BipolART

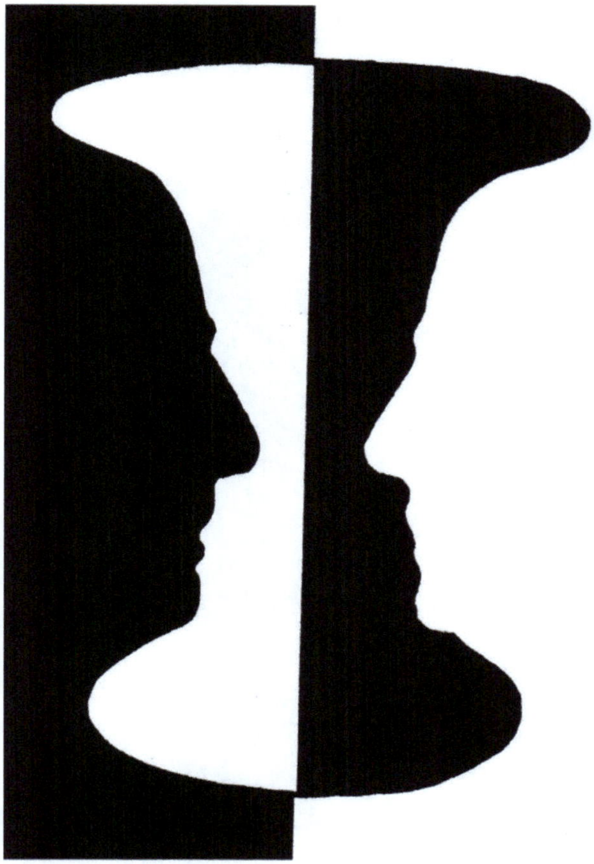

Denys N Wheatley

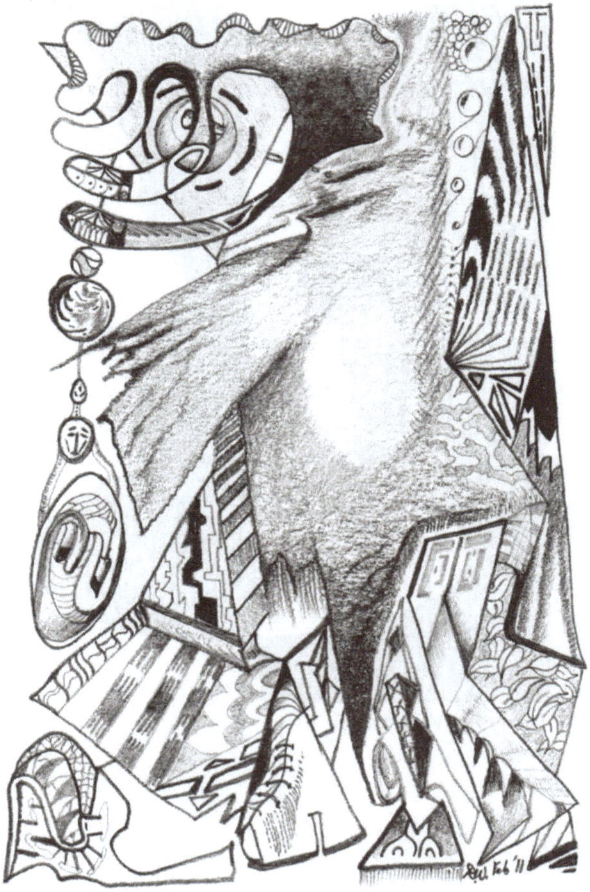

A typical late doodle (Yoyoscan, February 2011)

Denys N. Wheatley

"BipolART"

Art and Bipolar Disorder: A Personal Perspective

Springer

Dr. Denys N. Wheatley
BioMedES
Leggat House, Keithhall
Inverurie Aberdeenshire, AB51 0LX UK

ISBN 978-94-007-4871-2 ISBN 978-94-007-4872-9 (eBook)
DOI 10.1007/978-94-007-4872-9
Springer Dordrecht Heidelberg London New York

Library of Congress Control Number: 2012944647

Printed on acid-free paper

Springer is part of Springer Science + Business Media (www.springer.com)

Acknowledgements

To have written this book at my time of life, I am eternally grateful to my family, who have seen me through many long periods of depression, and at other times where I have been almost unmanageably manic. They must have suffered almost as much as myself in their way, but they have held me together such that I nevertheless could pursue a rewarding career in cancer research. I particularly want to thank my former wife, Pamela, my two daughters, Nina and Sally, and my present partner, Jean Fletcher.

I have been encouraged to write this book by a number of colleagues, some of whom know that I have bipolar disorder and others that are not so aware of my condition; they include Edward Mercer, Bhanu Jena, Reginald Goldacre, Ian Clark, and Lee Tsun Hou. There have been others, who—as artists themselves—saw that my efforts were not in vane; indeed they seem to indicate that I could have been something of an artist if I had chosen this as a career. These include Jennifer Jane Bayliss, Douglas Prosser, Bert Menco, Cynthia Coda, Jacqui Robertson and Marian Reid.

The Carnegie Trust of Scotland was generous in giving me an award as an emeritus staff of Aberdeen University to start this project. It would not have progressed much further if Springer (Dordrecht) had not also encouraged me after seeing my portfolio, and taken the bold step of offering a contract for the publishing of this book. Its content lies intentionally somewhere between science and art; it is neither a scientific/medical monograph nor an art book. Today we are seeing renewed and welcome activity in the interface between science and art, and how together they impact on society. I hope that my work will add a further small step in this direction.

Some of the paintings and drawings have been on show in local exhibitions, which has resulted in quite a number being purchased. Other pictures have been given to members of my family, whom I hope one day will see these works and the ones I will later leave as a tangible legacy. However, I cannot assume that the artwork will survive the test of time!

I also wish to acknowledge many of my newer friends whom I have made at the local mental health recovery centre. Together our art efforts have provided a focus for me, and a chance to share my work and feelings with them. There has been a long history of treatment with many doctors, psychiatrists, and clinical psychologists, whom I would like to pay tribute to their patience and helpful understanding of my condition. In particular, my recent GP, Dr. Hood and clinical psychologist, David Huxtable, has not only succeeded in getting me past cyclical depression, but saw the potential in the artwork in being incorporated into art therapy in future. I now have the task of finding out much more about the role of art therapy in mental disorders, for it is very apparent that we are all going to need much more help as we get older in keeping our brains and minds functioning in a healthy and focused manner. Once again, I reiterate the hope that what I have produced in this book can provide some insight into bipolar disorder such that its content can be assimilated in some way into the kinds of therapy that might work gently and humanely in lifting people out of the awful feelings of depression, and calm down those who are manic. To be creative in life, as we can all be, lifts our spirits and should make us happier in this stressful world that we seem to have inherited today.

Contents

List of Figures

Chapter 1
Prologue—By Way of an Introduction

No excellent soul is exempt from a mixture of madness.

Aristotle

It was not my original intention to say much up-front about what follows in the chapters of this book that are filled with artwork. The content should hopefully speak for itself, with a few short interjections helping to set the scene, or providing an apt quotation. The idea had been to let you wander through the "gallery" (the chapters of this book) first, and then for me to make some remarks about artwork and its therapeutic value in bipolar disorder, as well as a little about myself, in the Epilogue.

But the gallery needs some introduction, even if something about the person (personality) behind them is left until later. The artwork is an eclectic mixture of two-dimensional art produced over the last 12–13 years, although this is not the only phase during my life that manic-depression (bipolar disorder) has loomed large. The original idea of setting these works out in chronological order had to be abandoned since it proved better to collect them into groups, as can be seen from the chapter headings in the Contents, but deciding which picture went where was often difficult. Nevertheless I hope their presentation in this way works well.

There are simple pencil doodles in Chapter 2. Drawing them depends on who you are, and how you set about it is a personal matter. But in Chapter 3, I give a brief glimpse of how I build up some of the more abstract of them, and from there they could become very elaborate, as in Chapter 4. There is no doubt that doodles are almost always abstract, although many will contain images that are recognisable. Doodles in the last few years have, on average, become larger, as well as being more elaborate and stylised than before, a kind of new genre.

Some doodles have led to major paintings, although others were done without first drawing a doodle. A common motif can be seen in the many of the life-forms depicted in the early doodles, and therefore I have selected those which emphasis this aspect in Chapter 5 in a "biological journey". This is not surprising because of my biomedical training and background. The trend towards paintings rather than pencil doodles took off quite early, and many of them remain relatively true to life and nature; Chapter 6 is on "reality". A variety of different media have been used,

D. N. Wheatley, *BipolART*,
DOI 10.1007/978-94-007-4872-9_1,

and with them I have tried my hand at more "conventional subjects" (landscapes, buildings, people and flowers).

I also have a musical background and now live with a professional violinist. Since Jean and I got together, this has led to some doodles and paintings over the last 7 years that intentionally have a distinctly musical theme, giving me some relief and pleasure in doing something for someone very special as part of Art Therapy—you might even call it Music Therapy because we also play music together (Chapter 7).

Chapter 8 deals with one of my most interesting developments, with many larger, colourful abstract works. This is where I feel I can let myself go. A little later this is followed by an equally abstract room in the "gallery" that deals with geometrical form (Chapter 10). I have been interested in geometry to the point of obsession for many years, and in it triangles, circles, and spheres predominate. It is noteworthy that the "ideals" of Plato were spheres and triangles, so there is something very basic about them, and perhaps this may reflect quite considerably on my nature.

When not that depressed and in a more euthymic phase, I will be laughing, punning, cracking jokes and generally interacting comfortably with everyone else. A long time ago I became deeply interested in an exceedingly small and beautiful biological structure that can only be examined at the level of the electron microscope, called a "centriole". It has a triplet tubular structure with a quasi 9-fold symmetry; it is sometimes referred to as a pinwheel. On many occasions I have played with this natural design and tried to make humorous variations upon it. This has led to about 70–80 different variations on the basic structure, of which a selection is shown of some of the more amusing ones in Chapter 9. Many of them were done to pass the time on, for example, long-haul flights—perhaps to divert the mind from the work that had just been undertaken abroad (and perhaps a preventive against a possible lapse into depression on arriving home exhausted?). Doing this special type of doodling has always been fun, and a relief.

Chapter 11 is the Epilogue in which I will discuss mostly my personal views on the nature of bipolar as I see it, how I have felt and what impact this condition has overall on my life (and the life of others). The value of "doing", be it craft, music, gardening, etc., during depression is vitally important to recovery, and as I indicate from recent experience, it can also act in a preventive manner. I trust this will be of sufficient interest to help understand the condition, my dilemmas with it and what my art work might mean. Art cannot do other than express both conscious and subconscious feeling and images. I tend to think in pictures and therefore it is quite natural for me to express myself in this way.

A Little Background

While I was interested in art from a very young age, it was never going to be my career. Apart from a couple of courses lasting no more than a few hours or a day, I have received no formal training in art since leaving school. Being an inquisitive youngster, a passion for discovery eventually led me into a scientific career. Occasionally I enjoyed dabbling in art during a life-time's career in cancer research, but these turned out to be few and far between. The intensity and competitiveness of funding a busy research facility leaves little time (and energy) to pursue other activities.

At school in the 1950s, we were given the iniquitous choice between art and science streaming, which meant there was little development of my artistic skills from the end of "secondary 2" (about 13 years old). But scientists of my vintage were expected to draw innumerable specimens at school and university because of the "natural history" ethos of biological sciences that prevailed at that time. I found this relatively easy, and was good at memorising things, being fortunate enough to have something of an eidetic memory. This gave me a very useful talent in being able to draw something, for example, an animal such as a fox, from memory, and I have put this to good use in many of the my paintings and drawings.

I see no real division between Art and Science; such distinctions are man-made, not natural. My opinion, also held by others, is that creativity has much the same—almost indefinable—character wherever you meet it. If any difference exists, it is principally in that artistic expression is more *subjective,* an individual activity (at least with regard to painting and drawing), and a rather solitary affair, whereas creativity in the scientist, whilst emanating from the individual, claims to be more objective and related to others indulging themselves in similar analytical pursuits of Nature and the Universe that requires team-work and consensus, more so today than ever before.

Accepting that the pictures herein are by an amateur artist, they are the products of creativity mainly during episodes of depression in bipolar disorder. However, many of the bigger ones, especially the paintings, were completed when emerging from the worst weeks of the deepest low. Interestingly, very few drawings or paintings were started during manic and more euthymic periods of bipolar—there never seemed to be time to do so!

The images collected in this book are not for the art critic to weigh up (and perhaps trash), but are intended for those who have bipolar disorder (i.e. manic-depression[1]), and for others who may see art as an important therapeutic/remedial intervention. It is also intended for anyone taking an interest in this condition; indeed, I hope this includes the proverbial "man of the Clapham omnibus"—the layman. So I would hope that everyone can take an interest in the contents of this book, because we can all have mood swings. It just happens that some of us "swing" more extremely than others.

I have recently become aware of organizations that deal with art therapy within the field of mental strife, but have not so far directly involved myself with them. This

---

[1] As a scientist, I am trained to be particularly concerned about the precise meaning of words. With regard to the use of MD (manic-depression) and BP (bipolar disorder), the latter has now been adopted by the American Psychiatric Association and related societies, and is in widespread use. The former, however, has its place since many experts are of the opinion that MD is much more descriptive than BP. I will probably use both, for which I apologise. But this also raises another issue, that of the condition being a disorder, and one that had the stigma for many years of being a condition close to insanity. Since we all have the MD tendency, we also have to accept that we are talking about the more extreme cases in the wide spectrum of human behaviour.

may be a good thing in some ways, because I am following my own instinct, came to this activity myself, and was not (on reflection) wanting to be influenced by what others see as the beneficial aspects of the hands-on approach in times of mental stress. Readers may find interesting things in the pictures which tell them not only something about my psyche, but conjure up some impression in their own minds, i.e. reflect the viewer's psyche—especially those with similar or related mental conditions (e.g. schizophrenia). This begs the question—could these images be of any use in showing some features or manifestations commonly found in bipolar sufferers? For me, the therapy works in many ways as one form of catharsis, but it is used alongside a familiar range of interventions that bipolar sufferers are given -tranquillizing drugs, lithium, rest, steady exercise, regular long walks, meditation, group therapy, electro-convulsive therapy, among other things.

You will find that I shall be asking questions like this at several places throughout the book. While questions need answers, the rhetorical ones should at least set your thinking and cogitating on the images they portray (what you see in them).

Another issue I want to raise at the start is that I have no reasons for drawing this collection together other than those just mentioned. Although Springer kindly gave me a contract so that I could express my *self* (sic) in this way, it has not been done for any personal (financial) gain, but for others to see what has come out of one sufferer's mind. If I should find myself in receipt of any royalties, these will be given to a charity concerned with mental health and the removal of its stigma in society that thankfully is beginning to be expunged. Given its increasing frequency in society, especially the young (discussed in the Epilogue), it will have far less stigma when more and more people admit to mood swings and mental disorders in our future increasingly competitive world where the average age in the population is also increasing because most of us are living a decade or more longer.

I have read many books on manic depression and others devoted solely to depression. A lot of them are personal accounts. Indeed, there are many more about depression (monopolar) than about the bipolar type. But there is one further and very important reason for producing this book. It is because all accounts I have come across have almost certainly *not* been written when the person was in deep despair (the pits) or extreme mania, but during a more "normal" (euthymic) phases, i.e. when they were neither too elated nor too dejected. However, Andrew Solomon indicated that he might have attempted to write when very depressed, and that even after recovering, he still found it a problem over the next 5 years—during which he amassed an enormous amount of information and insight from painstaking research of the literature:

> Writing on depression is painful, sad, lonely and stressful.
>
> (Andrew Solomon: *The Noonday Demon*)

Whilst it is more likely that writing about depression in the euthymic or manic phases can be more coherent, it seems to me utterly impossible that anyone can write "lucidly" about their condition from a subjective point of view when actually experiencing the worst nightmares of a depressive trough. There is seldom if ever the motivation or the energy to do so at such times, and the concentration span is far too short to write anything that is coherent or significant, especially when the memory also becomes appallingly bad. It is difficult to find the right words, unless one was more like one of the melancholic poets that seemed to convey the dreadful feelings, images and thoughts that pervade a sufferer. Dryden seemed to wallow in sadness:

> I strongly wish for what I faintly hope;
> Like the daydreams of melancholy men,
> I think and think on things impossible,
> Yet love to wander in that golden maze
> (John Dryden: *Rival Ladies*)

Almost all accounts are therefore written *retrospectively*, when the worst mood has passed, in the hope that the words can still recall and communicate some of the feelings of the mind in the torments of despair that might have been recently experienced. But the pain of deep depression is difficult to recall after the event, much like the pain of childbirth. In truth, it is also very difficult to find words that connote and can convey those dark thoughts, the mood and the utter despair experienced in the worst troughs of bipolar.

> Sometimes when I wrote I was a bit down, sometimes I was high and sometimes I was even higher up than that and so different versions of me have contributed to this book.
> (Brian Adams: *The pits and the pendulum*)

My contention is that if I doodle, sketch and paint when I am actually in the pits, then at least I am "recounting" something about my inner state *at the time*, and not *after* the event. I do not want to go into further historical and clinical details about my life and the bipolar disorder upfront, but will add some relevant comments in the "Epilogue". And there is one further highly relevant point that has been made by other authors who have BP. It is a condition that few people truly understand unless they have personally experienced it in all its severity, both up and down.

What I prefer is for you first to take "a walk through the gallery" in which each chapter is a different room with usually a different overall theme. I would prefer you also to resist the temptation to turn to the last chapter, like a reader of a "who-done-it", to find out more about the personality behind them before seeing what the art seems to portray in and of itself. But before starting out, I should add a few general comments on art in bipolar disorder.

Art and Therapy

It would be inappropriate to leave out a bit about art (all forms of art, from music to crafts) and its role in therapy, as far as I see things from my point of view. In brief, I will consider three of the main benefits that might be gained. To do anything first requires an *idea* in the mind, and enough motivation to take some action. A doodle—starting with a squiggle—is not really much of an idea, indeed it is simplicity itself; it should be a spontaneous activity. However, it follows from the old adage "even the longest journey starts with a single step" that a squiggle on a page is something external and tangible, and represents a "start". It has to go somewhere, and so it becomes embellished (Chapter 4). Small hints—perhaps in minutes, several hours, or even days afterwards—arise as to what the doodle might include or where it might go next, and so on until a momentum is built up in time that can take it through many stages of development. In the early doodles, very little time was spent over them, but they would hint of something and be soon completed in some semi-recognisable form.

The second benefit is that, as this process gets going, the *concentration* span increases and improves quite dramatically as the usual self-correcting phase of recovery gains pace. Finally, there becomes a need to achieve a more complete image, bringing true focus, purpose and a real goal into play—the mind goes on creating a firmer image of what the final product ought to be, and self-esteem rises as things move towards completion. As the doodling bug took me, this led to many complex pictures that required quite a long time to build up. There is also the comforting feeling of having achieved something, however seemingly trivial. Everything is the expression of one's inner self, and others might see in it a reflection of their own moods, emotions, and healthy (or unhealthy) disposition. The exercise can be (should be) truly cathartic in this respect; it is a *positive* act and definitely better than harping on negative and destructive thoughts. It is also the expression of an emotional state that is difficult to achieve through direct interaction with other people, usually shunned during deep depression. As one emerges from depression, the ability to cope with and relate to other people increases, but that is after the storm has really subsided and need not concern us here.

> O hateful error, melancholy's child!
> Why dost thou show,
> To the apt thoughts of men,
> The things that are not.
> (Shakespeare: *Julius Caesar*; v, iii, l.67)

I hope that other people might, through some form of (or formal) psychological analysis, such as using the Rorschach Inkblot Test, be able to see how art in itself is a cry, often a desperate attempt, to communicate with others, for mind has been called, and almost certainly is, a social phenomenon. Without human interaction, the vast majority of us would soon become mad. Interestingly, art work is used for people who have disordered thought processes or cannot emotionally communicate their feeling, emotion and ideas with their family, friends and strangers. Some will continue their dabbling in art in small groups of similar sufferers who come together with the help of caring professions skilled in helping people with a wide range of mental aberrations. We are gregarious animals, and need the encouragement, guidance and help of others, both our peers and those who have committed their professional lives to caring for the well-being of the oppressed in mind, in whatever form it is manifest. And this is most needed when in the depths of depression.

Art work should become a continuing activity that fends off impending depression, i.e. it can be a preventive measure. Finally, and hopefully, this book will be of some use to psychologists, psychiatrists, and other professionals who take a greater interest in a mental health problem that has for too long been stigmatised.

> Art is non-verbal communication that can reveal deeper emotions and insights.
>
> (Emma Mansfield: *The Little Book of the Mind*)

Most pictures (especially the bigger ones) will have the following information below them, only the right-hand information in bold being shown:

Title: **Palm tree in Madeira**
Medium: **Watercolour**
Date: **February 2003**
Size (w x h in cm): **14 x 9**

Chapter 2
Doodles—From the Beginning

Demonic frenzy, moping melancholy, and moon-struck madness
(Milton: *Paradise Lost-* a remarkably apt and succinct description of manic depression)

The beginning for me was the year 1998 when, during an episode of severe depression, I began to doodle, which I had previously never done, as I thought. I just took to my bed in a catatonic "trance" that overwhelms one in depression. Sporadic indulgence in art during a scientific career, apart, this is when art became much more meaningful for me as a regular activity to help with depressive phases, and subsequently as a preventive measure.

Within a few weeks, this doodling had become a habit and a focus that started to get me "out of myself"—that dark den into which one retreats when depressed, shunning the world and lacking any motivation to do anything, see anyone, and accomplish even the most trivial task.

> Manic-depression distorts moods and thoughts, incites dreadful behaviours, destroys the basis of rational thought, and too often erodes the desire and will to live.
> (Kay Redfield Jamison; *An unquiet mind*)

I start with a collection of these early doodles. In the years since that time, it was not unusual that a bigger work of art began to take shape from a doodle, even if it always started from just a continuous squiggle on a blank page. Doodling requires nothing other than a sheet of paper and a pencil or pen. It requires no training, and the interesting thing is that the outcome is mostly unpredictable. It develops rather than tries to capture a specific image that one has retained in the mind, as many a professional artist would do. This, in its simple way, begins to help in unravelling some of the agitation, confusion and conflicts existing in the mind of the depressed person.

I mentioned in the Prologue that I had done very little art throughout my career, except for a series of drawings and paintings done between 1968 and 1970 in the USA. In reviewing some of the anatomical drawings I had done at college, a small piece of green graph paper (as was used in 1959) fell out, and I was quite astonished to see that it was a doodle, no doubt done during a lecture. It was entitled "Writer's world" (the doodle below), but I cannot remember doing it or having any reason for

D. N. Wheatley, *BipolART*,
DOI 10.1007/978-94-007-4872-9_2, © Springer Science+Business Media Dordrecht 2012

this subject. This was not followed up until 1998, and I cannot say that I was usually an avid doodler during lectures, or when, for example, having a long conversation of the telephone. But there was a beginning, and in college I had two manic episodes and two depressions every year. At that time I struggled through the depressions and tried to hide my condition, making up for my poor performance during depression by furiously working during the manic phases, only to exacerbate the cycle until later I had to receive clinical treatment in my twenties.

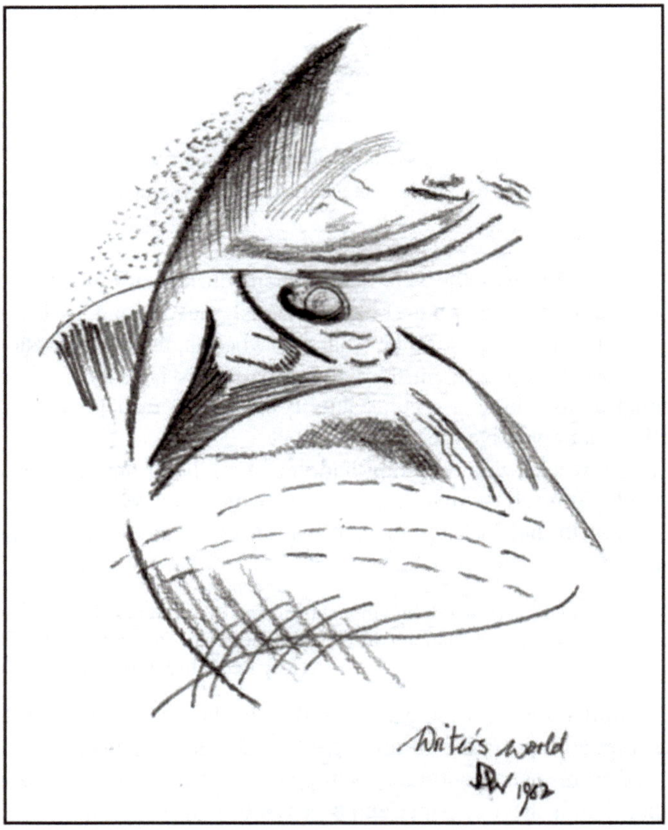

I started to doodle in November 1998, and I must have completed 40 doodles in a period of 2–3 months of depression during the winter of 1998–1999. Most were simple doodles, drawn in perhaps 15 minutes, sometimes with a vague object in mind as the first lines were drawn that soon took on a semblance of some real image, and definitely so in the next picture (with its remark at the top revealing my condition).

The next eight pictures in pencil each fit neatly on A4 pages. The first six were done in the depression of winter 1998. More often after a few random lines that started a doodle, it would begin to suggest something vaguely recognizable that I had no preconceived, such as a skirt or an old table leg, although the "finished product" was seldom a familiar object. Few of them were scribbled doodles; they are mostly tidy, usually with clear outline forms with quite sparse shading. This contrasts with how I later set about doodling (as demonstrated in the next chapter), especially more recently (2010/2011) in producing those found at the end of Chapter 4.

From the start, I have had the habit of giving each doodle a title that indicated the object or mood it seemed to resemble.

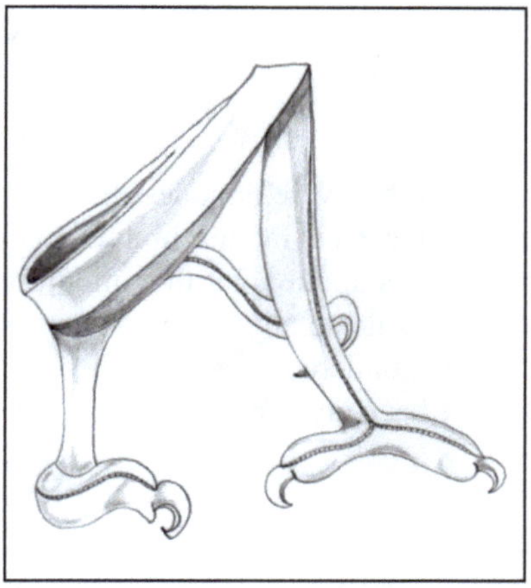

Grip stand

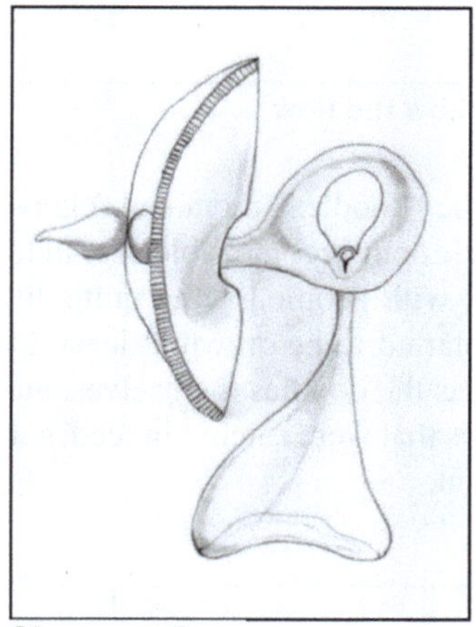

Glassy eardrop

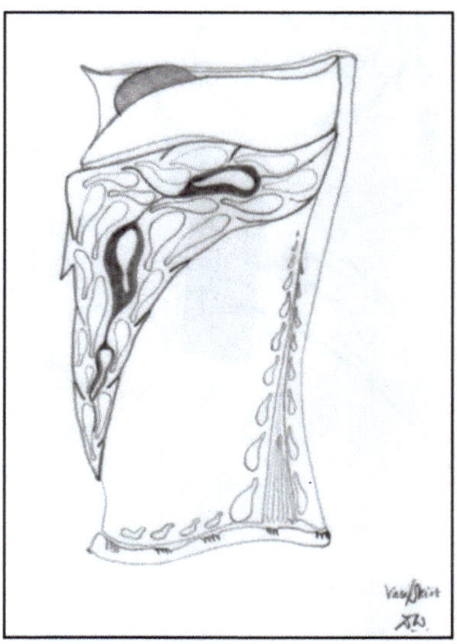

Vase/skirt

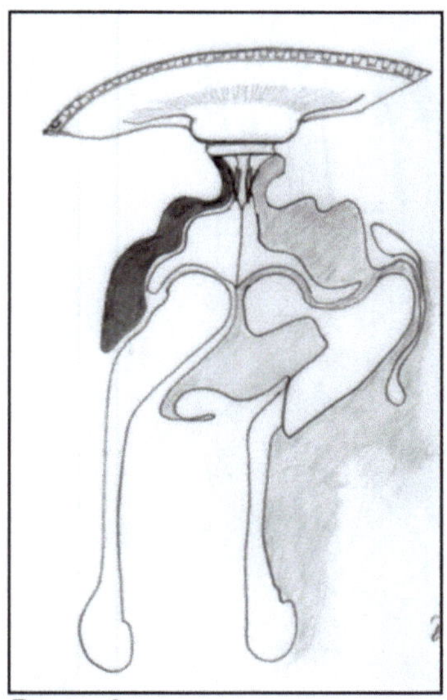

Draped urn

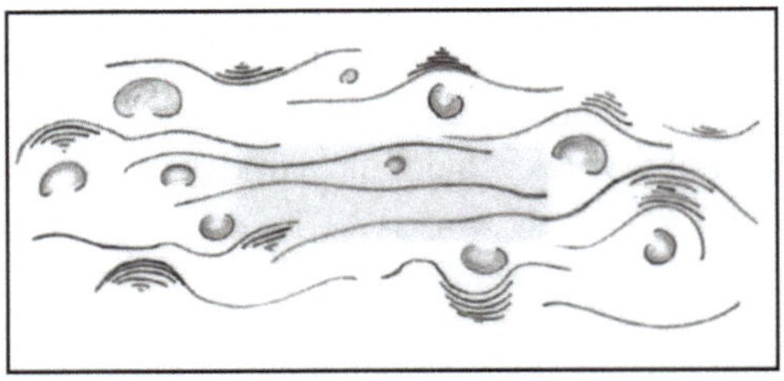

Follow the flow

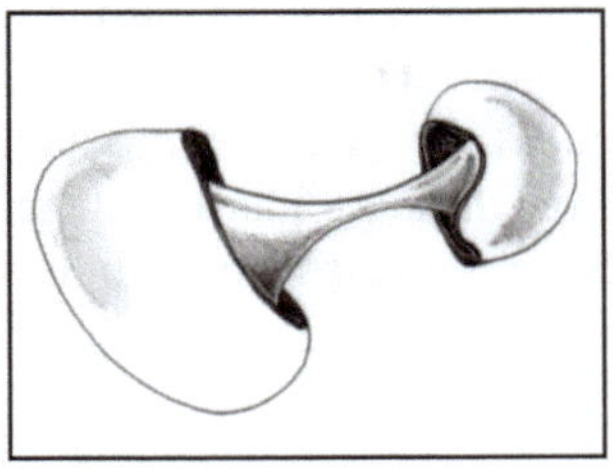

Full swivel

Later, the "doodles" remained relatively small, but were done less hurriedly. These have little or no recognizable overall form or subject, but include hints of recognizable objects, with people having quite different ideas about what they might represent. These started to be drawn at least 2 years after those above. The names can be as bizarre as the doodles themselves, and I often pondered for some time over them to find ones that were catchy; indeed, some have been given names that I have invented, e.g. Frent.

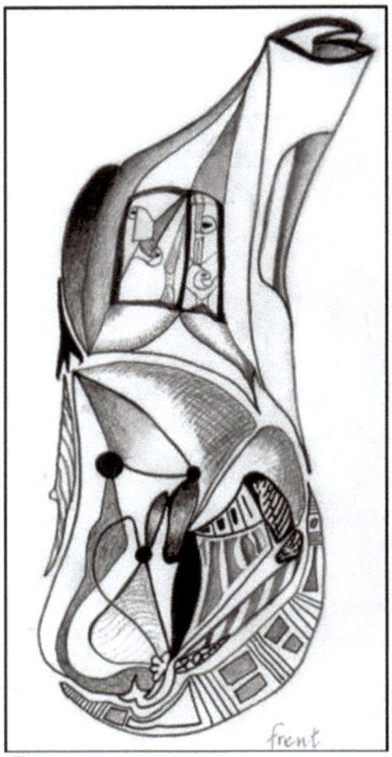

Frent
Pencil
January 2011
9 x 14

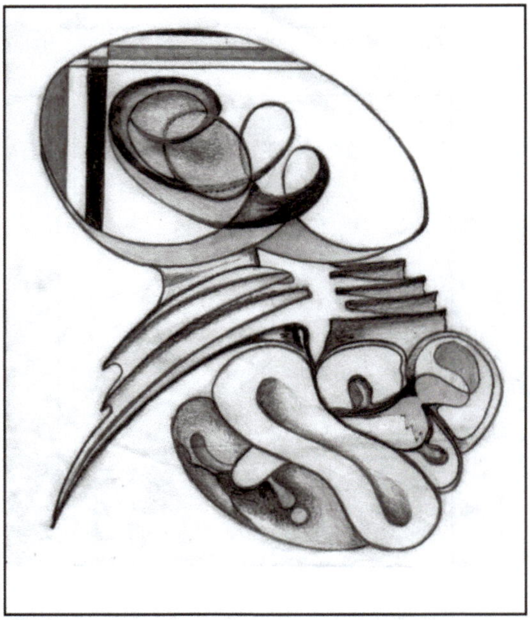

Clot
Pencil
December 2006
12 x 13

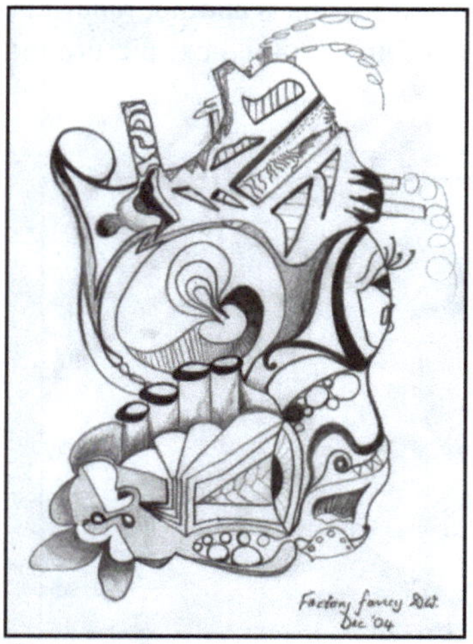

Factory fancy
Pencil
December 2004
10 x 16

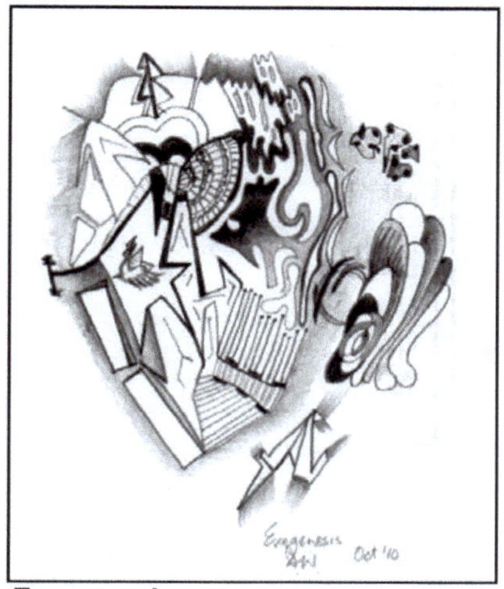

Exegenesis
Pencil
October 2010
11 x 11

Soon drawings started to become larger and took longer still than 15 minutes, sometimes a day or more, on and off; but these are nothing compared with the bigger doodles that came later.

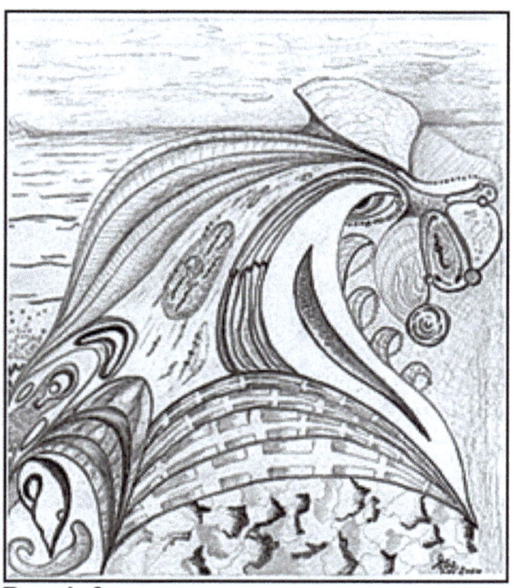

Beach forms
Pencil
November 2004
17 x 16

The one above has the sea as a background, and oddly this is another recurrent theme has turned up many times over the years of doddling, as the next picture indicates, here with mountains.

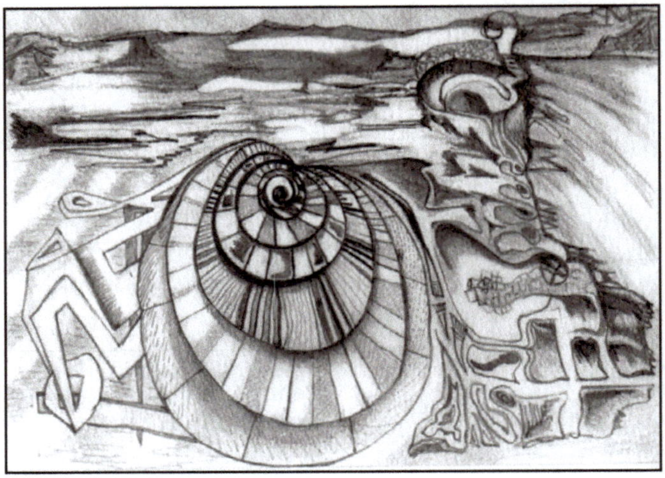

Beach scene
Pencil
January 2006
16 x 26

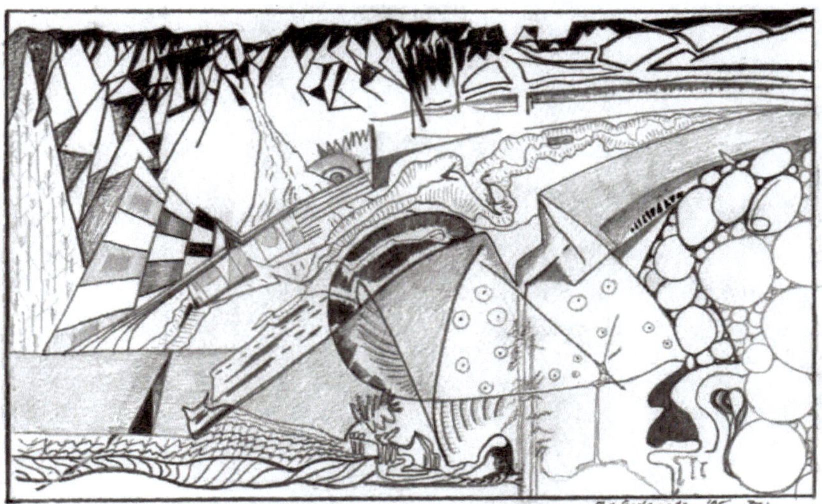

Old Esplanade
Pencil
February 2005
24 x 15

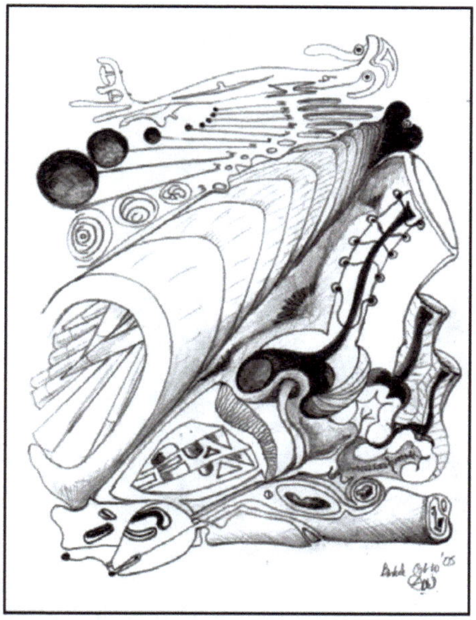

Bankok
Pencil
October 2005
11 x 16

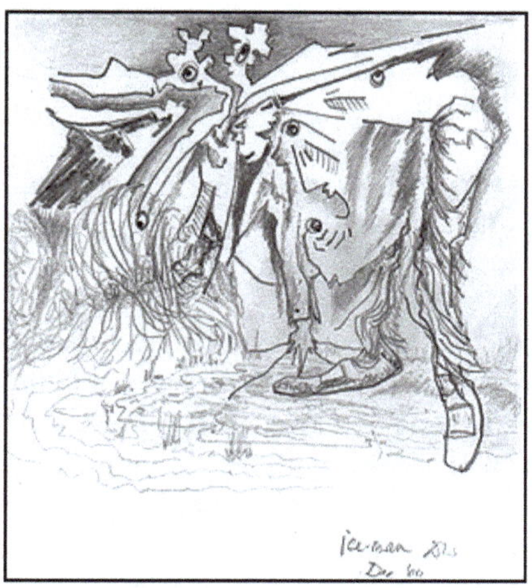

Ice-man
December 2006
Pencil
12 x 13

Many of the doodles started to get that they would not fit easily on to A4 sheets, on which most previous images had been drawn.

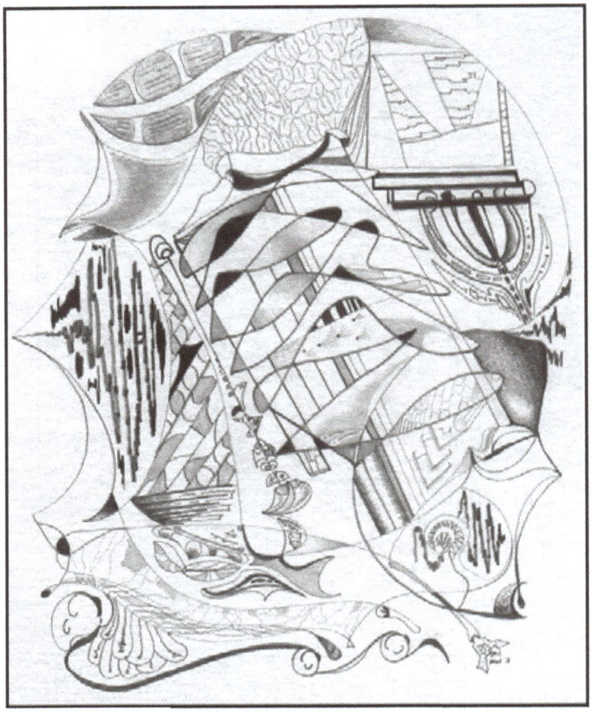

Headache
Pencil
March 2011
21 x 24

It is odd that the doodle below developed into a very formal evocation of the motif of the two fishes representing Pisces. Once it had got to this stage, it had to be done for my grandson, who, like me, is a Piscean. It is ironic that the yin-yang of Pisces is the sign of the Zodiac that accords with my own bipolar temperament. Some might see this as "destiny", not without meaning in realms of which we may currently have no knowledge; but I just see it simply as a coincidence. The second image is a play on the yin-yang motif, which would also make an apt logo for BP. But it also harps back to a doodle earlier in this chapter at the top of page 12.

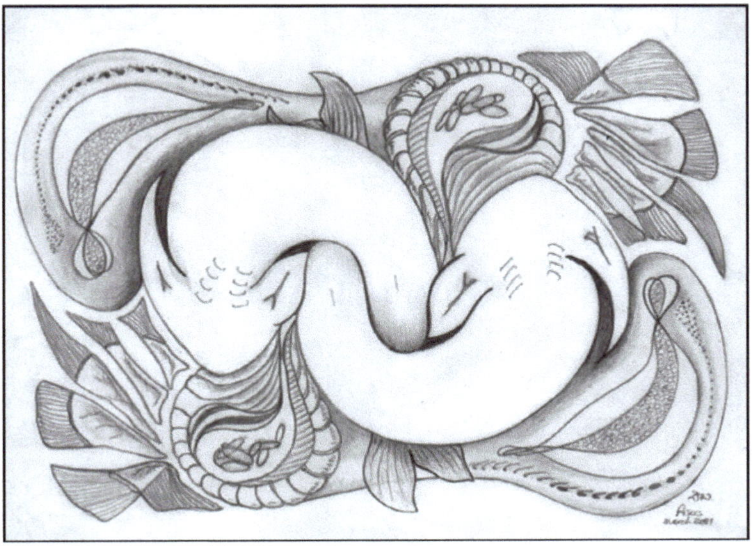

Pisces
March 2001
Pencil
28 x 19

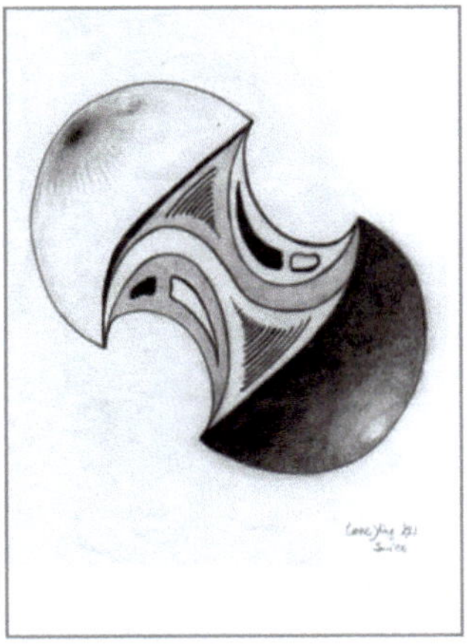

Core yin-yang
Pencil
January 2006
10 x 12

Chapter 3
Drawing Doodles

Nothing could be simpler than doodling. You need a surface that you can draw on—a piece of paper—and something to draw with, a pencil, a piece of charcoal, or a crayon. And then you just let anything happen—spontaneous drawing! I am probably too conventional, but the surface is usually stiff white paper so that it is easy to draw on it almost anywhere, with no need for an easel, a desk or a table. (Modern devices allow us to use iPads and similar machines for doodling, but I personally do not find using computers for producing art-work satisfying, for which I can give no particular reason. If David Hockney can produce a massive amount of work on an iPad that is as appealing as any of his more conventional earlier works, then clearly it is a good method for those to whom it does appeal.)

If we look at the next images, the one on the left started with a series of detached squiggles on a page of A3 before taking off. So the lines on the doodle on the left became integrated and created the doodle on the right. A definite idea

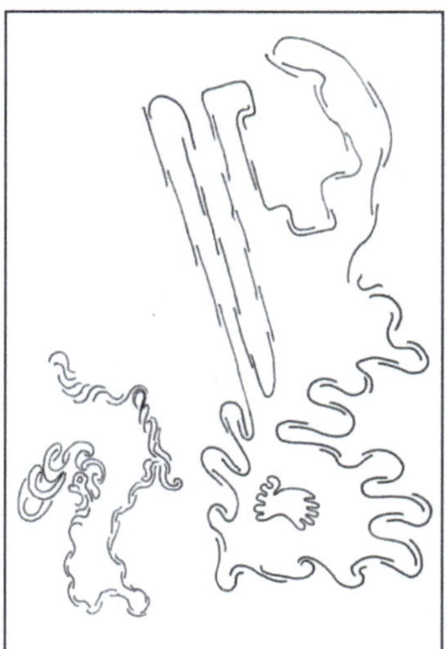

Starting doodle
Pencil
November 1998
28 x 40

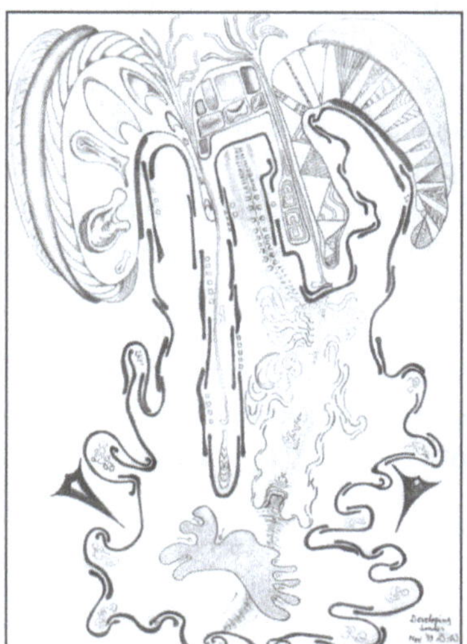

Developing senses (final doodle)
Pencil
November 1998
28 x 40

D. N. Wheatley, *BipolART*,
DOI 10.1007/978-94-007-4872-9_3, © Springer Science+Business Media Dordrecht 2012

took over and the image began to look like an outline of the development of the nervous system in the body, with bulging eye-like structures (reminiscent of the hugely disproportionate eyes of a young chick embryo). This example gives you some idea how far a few lines can go once you get started.

I will deal with a few simpler doodles, following the steps by which they were constructed.

First Example

My doodles usually start with pencil lines on a firm piece of white board on my lap. *Step 1* is to make a squiggle with a soft (2B) pencil, usually taking no more than a few seconds. It is deliberately set out here as a random line, with no particular subject or objective in mind, which is in many ways freer that the first doodles shown in Chapter 2, where each very soon led to an end result that had more than a passing similarity to some familiar object.

I had little idea where I was going with the first line, except to ensure it was kept reasonably central on the paper. I recommend this way of starting because it does not matter how big or small the piece of paper is, or how extensive the first lines are made. Next comes a slightly different task; you probably want to put another squiggle over or beside the first one, but sometimes I start to think a bit more about developing (i.e. joining up) bits of the first squiggle, as in *step 2*. Every time something is added, new ideas might come to mind, many of these floating somewhere between the subconscious and conscious levels. *Step 2* seems to suggest a couple of fingers, but I was certainly was not trying to produce this image, and this idea—even if it did register at the time—was not taken any further, so I still had no notion where this doodle was leading me.

The doodle looks very barren as simple lines, and it seemed time to start adding some embellishments. In the next step (*step 3*), some claws, teeth or spikes (could be any of these), with curved veils below them, were added, but I don't know why. Most of the drawing seemed to be on the right-hand side of the doodle, and being a person who prefers balance and a semblance of symmetry, my next move (*step 4*) was to add new material on the left-hand side. In contrast to the right-hand side, I added mostly straight lines, but I am not sure that this was done intentionally. The lines started to join up some of the floppy ends of the original squiggle. Little infills were also being added (solid black and light grey areas, done with 3B and 2H pencils, respectively).

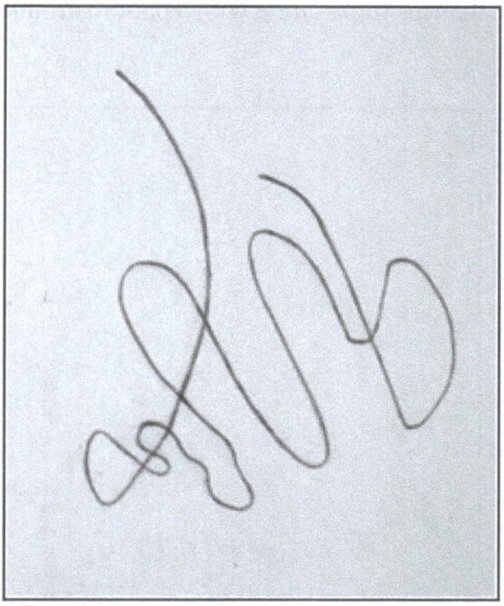

Step 1

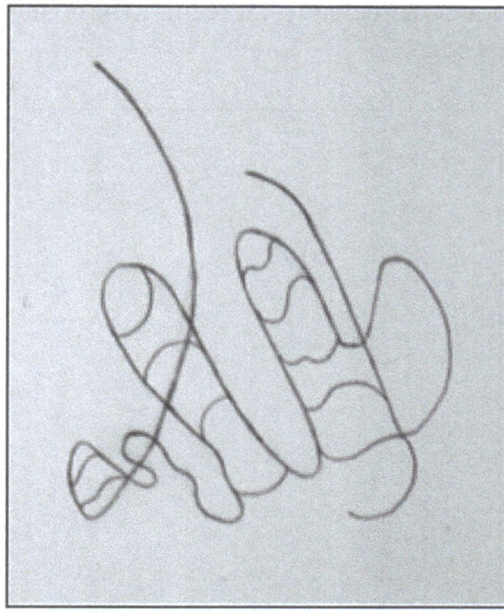

Step 2

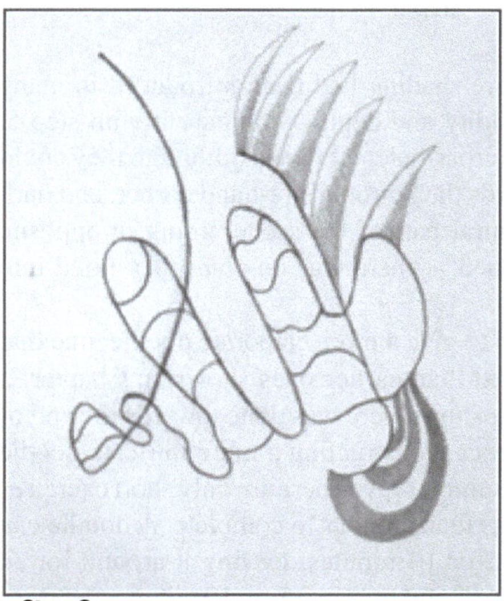

Step 3

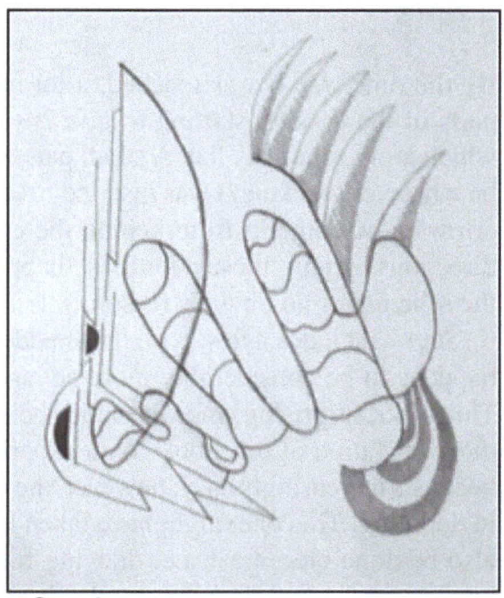

Step 4

Things were now "taking shape", which is paradoxical because the whole idea of a doodle is that it is not supposed to be representative of anything in particular. However, it does begin to acquire a form of its own that seems to direct the artist towards an end-point that can consolidate the overall pattern. All sorts of motifs seemed to be emerging, and some no doubt would be chosen in my mind that would help develop the doodle. On the right-hand side in *step 5*, an eye-like image was included, as if partly hidden behind the original loop in that area. I do not think it was intentionally drawn as an eye; in other words, I have no recollection that it was done "deliberately". It seems to be no more than a simple circle with a pattern around its edge.

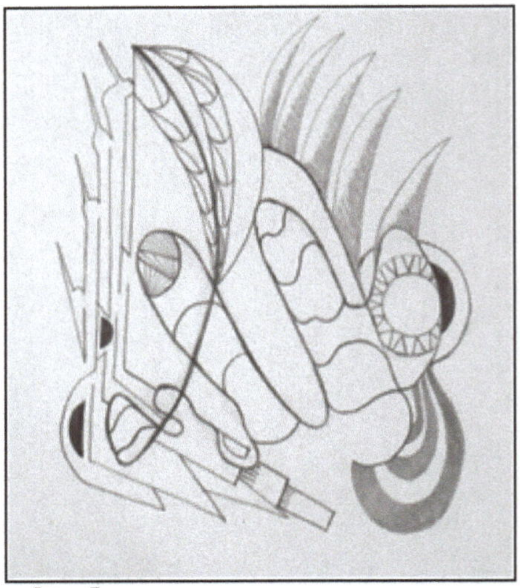

Step 5

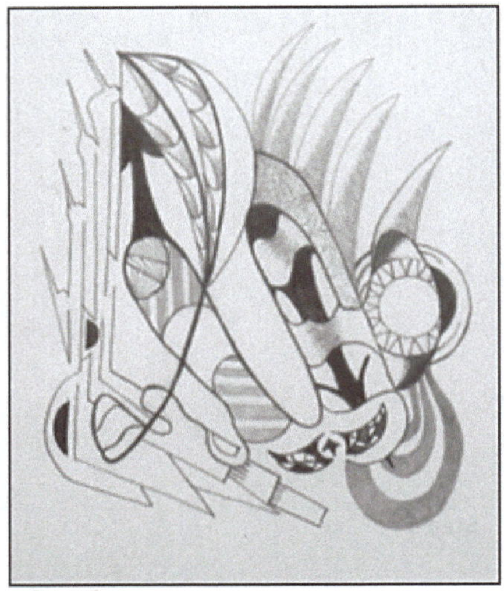

Step 6

By the time *step 6* was reached, a lot more shading had been introduced in many parts of the doodle, starting to give it solidity and depth—compare it with step 5, which looks relatively flat. A small pair of cross-hatched wings (although they could be whatever you fancy) was inserted towards the bottom right-hand corner, and dark arrows now come in from behind the central part of the scene, going in opposite directions. Again, these additions "happened"—there was no plan; they fitted into the scheme for no obvious reason.

Step 7 includes a few extra items added to give a more elaborate doodle, one that happens to be considerably more advanced than earlier ones shown in Chapter 2. This is not surprising since the series being shown here was done towards the end of the preparation of this book. With experience, constructing a more intricate doodle becomes increasingly easy; however, the examples given here are only short exercises in doodling. This one might have taken less than an hour to complete. A doodle can also be done piecemeal, i.e. drawing for 5 or 10 minutes, leaving it around for an hour or a day, and then coming back to it to add another 5 or 10 minutes work to it, perhaps several times. One way or another, a doodle carries on evolving until it seems to have gone far enough. Like so many things in life, the problem more often than not is to know when to stop, to leave it alone and let it assume its own existence. From *step* 7 on to *step 8*, a few more finishing touches have been added until that moment came when it seemed quite clear that the end product had been reached. In step 7, for example, there is a curvaceous dotted structure around and contrasting with the spiky pieces, like a background drape. Adding it seemed to pull the doodle together at the top—clearly there was a quite firm intention in what was being done rather than adding a new feature such as another random agglomeration

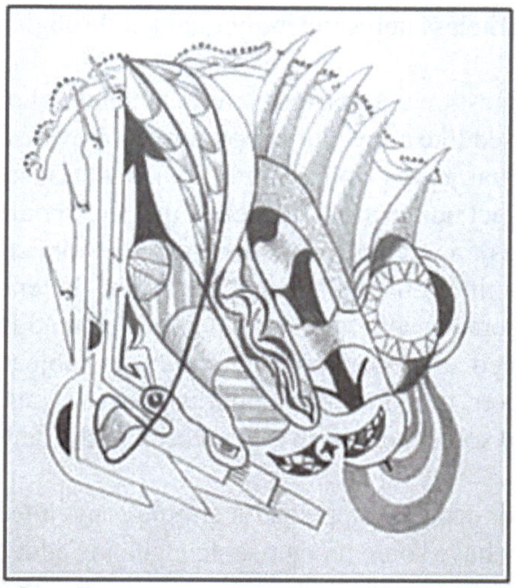

Step 7

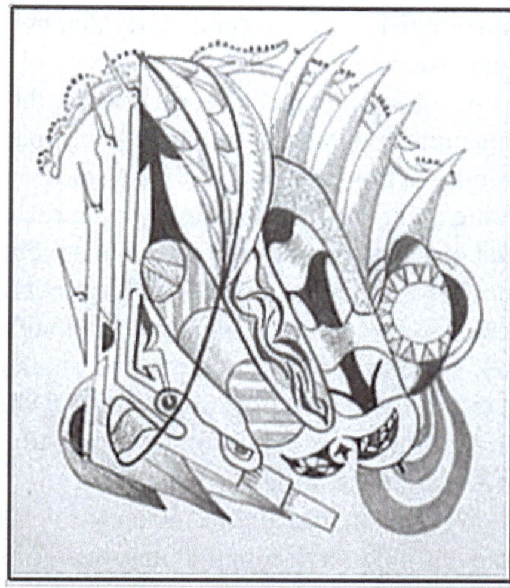

Step 8

of squiggles. The finishing touch in step 8 is hardly noticeable—little more than light shading of the sharp bits in the bottom left-hand corner. This gave a few white areas more depth and substance, suggesting there had been a definite intent to make them something more "solid" by not just gratuitously adding a flat in-fill. As this example shows, it becomes increasingly more difficult to add anything to a doodle in a truly random fashion. The doodle at some point takes on its own character, usually when it nearer completion.

The question might be asked as to whether the drawing represents "a work of art" to be kept, or just a pile of scribbling on a piece of paper to be screwed up and thrown into the waste basket. When doodling is done while listening to someone on the telephone, a common practice (on which subject, more in the Epilogue), the result often turns out to be some recognizable form, but it is usually small, crammed on to the edge of a notepad or newspaper, and will almost certainly be trashed. But a person who is mentally disturbed doing a doodle of the type just illustrated will probably not see the result at step 8 as just a bit of rubbish. It will be the product of that person's mind and imagination, no matter how random the work might seem. Returning some time later to a doodle after it has come into an existence of its own, it is not uncommon for the artist (in this case myself) to have little or no recollection of doing it (especially during depression). It has become something separate from the self, but nevertheless with hidden connections that can run quite deep. One can also see something different in it each time it is viewed. Furthermore, other people will see and "interpret" your doodle in totally different ways. Herein lies the fascination of doodling; it cannot help but give some insight into the mind of the artist, both as a personal reflection, and as a statement that others can see and respond to accordingly as they might wish. Thus it also reflects the viewer's mind! To me, it follows that it is a useful form of communication that allows one to interact with the world, but it can as easily be a covent activity that nevertheless helps the individual get through a depression.

Assuming others can see a doodle, the question that intrigues me is whether art of this quite spontaneous nature can be analysed like conventional paintings by critical minds (in this case psychologists and psychiatrists as well as art critics), and has any value other than the seemingly cathartic effect on the artist. It is clear that the doodle that has just been developed is not a picture of a recognizable object or set of objects that took shape in a predictable (predetermined) manner. For this reason, the end result should have no meaning (although some cryptic message(s) might be read in it!). On this account, it cannot be challenged as a poor representation of a subject. It either *looks good* or it does not—whatever, that does not matter, since it was the doing of it that was important, especially to someone otherwise "locked" in the dark recesses of the mind.

What, then, has all this meant to the BP or depressed person? A simple convoluted line has led to a design that may seemingly have some recognisable elements added to it, such as teeth, arrows and eyes. And yet none of this bizarre collection is ever likely to be seen together in real life. The imagination has been at work, and has externalised associations made somewhere the brain. It has led to something which is interesting, different and, in particular, unique. And anyone can do it! Some skill is needed at times, such as knowing how to shade, but the best way to make doodles is simply to start doodling, and then go on and on doodling. If nothing else, the activity is relaxing, just like spinning yarn or weeding a garden is supposed to be.

To anyone in deep depression, doodling can be a useful form of therapy. For some of us, it might become habitual, leading on to it becoming a very stylized and formal kind of art, as seen in Chapter 4 and beyond. The images were the result of my fascination with what was emerging as time went by over the years, and I resorted to this practice whenever I fell into a deep depression. Latterly, as mentioned above, I have started doodling *before* becoming depressed rather than leaving things until I have reached the pits. It is too early to say whether it has helped since I have only done this over the last 2 years. Its contribution will be difficult to assess because I have been doing this more diligently along with other strategies designed to ward off impending BP depressive episodes.

A Second Example

The next example of creating a doodle is equally simple, if not simpler, than the first. It shows that no matter how you start, you might end up with something similar to the first lines or something quite different. In reviewing a large collection of doodles produced over 12–13 years, I wonder if anyone might find a unifying theme. Would someone looking at many of them know that it was the same person who produced them, just as one can recognize a Monet or a van Gogh ? This does not seem to ring true if we believe the notion that every doodle is largely random and unique. A degree of contrivance might have entered consistently into doodles drawn over many years.

There can often be a remarkable similarity between doodles done several years apart, with some form of subconscious recollection at work, which can be quite uncanny (as will be shown in Chapter 10 on geometry). Do the recurrent forms indicate any particular "aberration" or obsession in my brain? Be that as it may, let us see the second doodle develop. It does have some similarities in the early stages of the first doodle in this chapter, but then it diverges to give an increasingly different result, and once again it cannot be likened to any recognizable object in life. It also led in this case to the use of colour to brighten it up—black and white pencil drawings can sometimes become boring! *Steps 1–6* in this second example show a series of simple "waves" that are progressively linked up with bands. Shading again gives added perspective, especially going from steps 6 to 7. And then colour was used in *steps 8 and 9*, giving the whole design extra appeal, with eight being better than nine, but that's a personal preference regarding the colours used. To do these last two images, photocopies were made of step 6, and these were coloured individually with crayons. I called it "skelter" at this stage (helter skelter?).

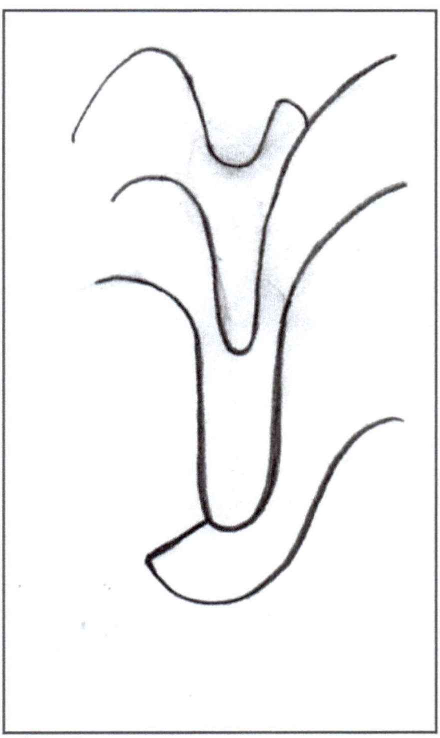

Step 1

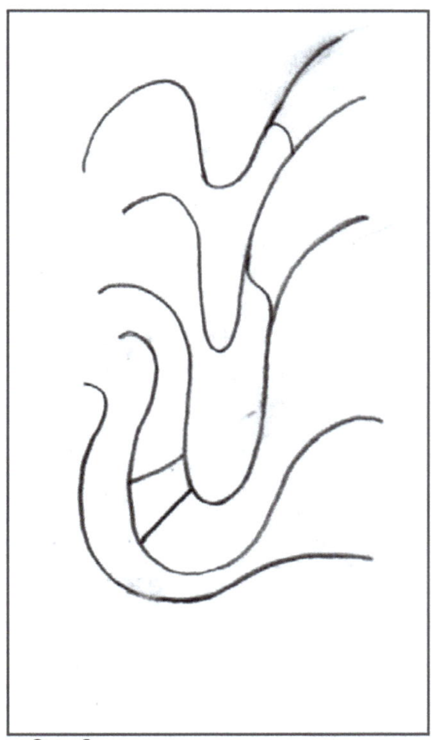

Step 2

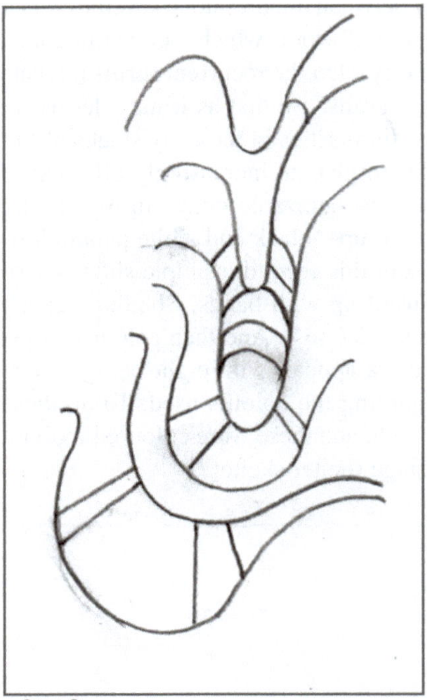

Step 3

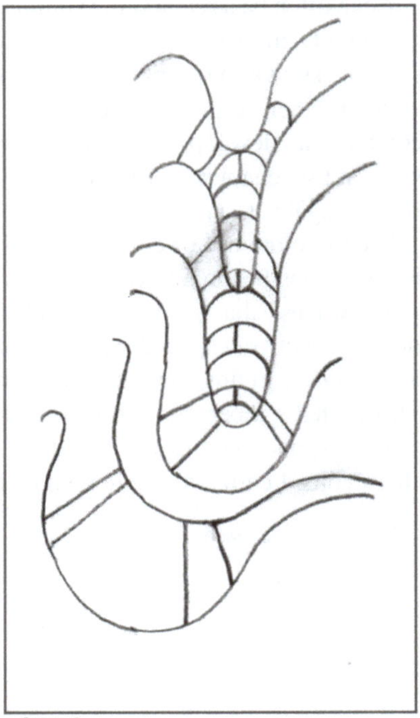

Step 4

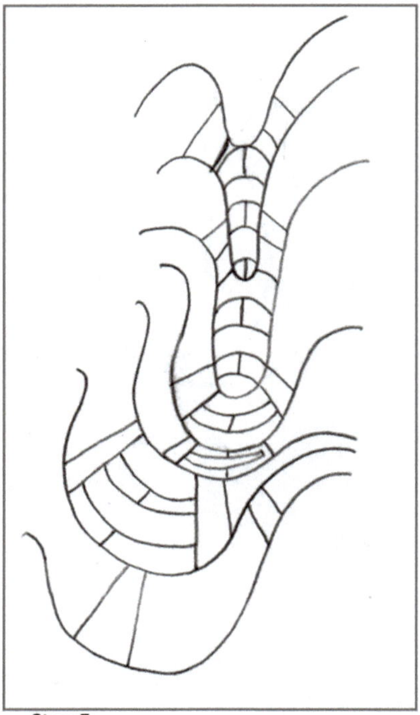

Step 5

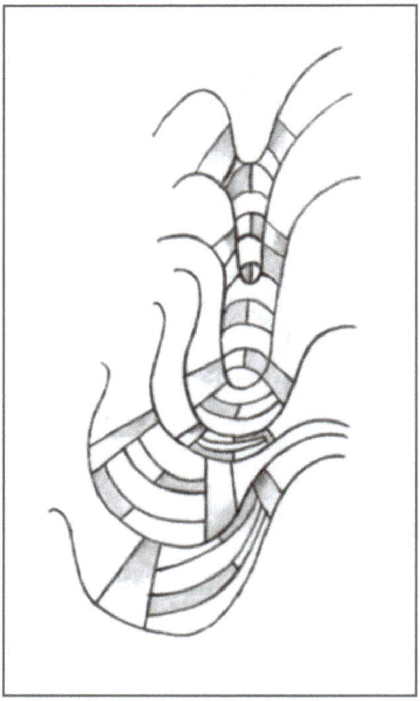

Step 6

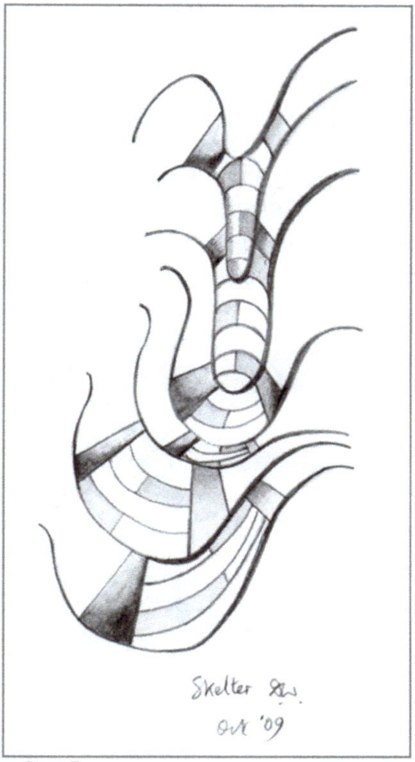

Step 7

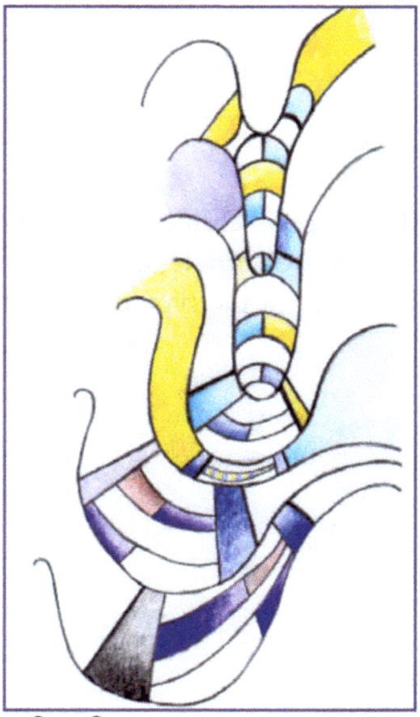

Step 8

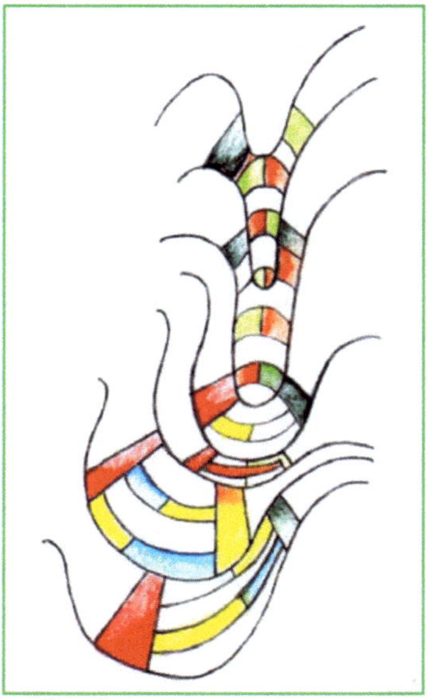

Step 9

Where Doodling Might Take You?

In an uncanny way once again, the characters of these two sets of doodles somehow resonated in my mind after I had done them, and resulted in a hybrid of the coloured doodle seen in step 9 immediately above and the more pointed features in the first set of doodles. The colours were carefully considered to get them to blend together within the different areas of the doodle. Anything goes in doodling, so do not over-conceptualise what you are doing—just do it.

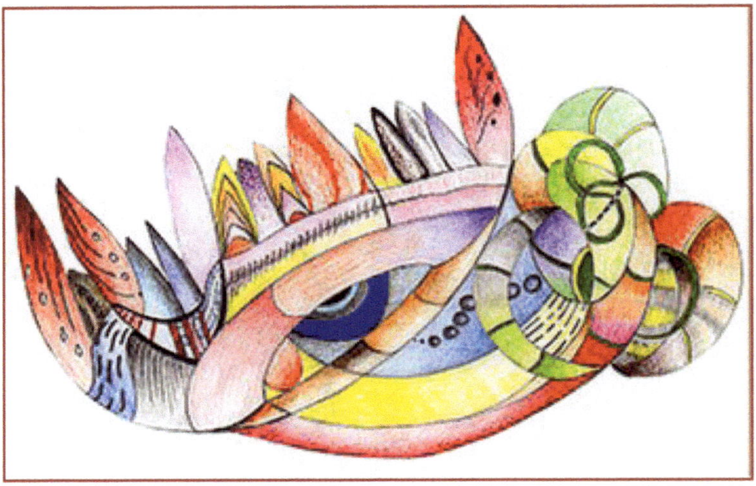

Crab-clawed
Crayon and Pencil
December 2010
15 x 12

But the next is in great contrast—a doodle of considerable size (A3), in which I got carried away, ending up with something highly elaborate that would have taken many hours to complete (rarely at one sitting), and of the type that will be seen in the next chapter.

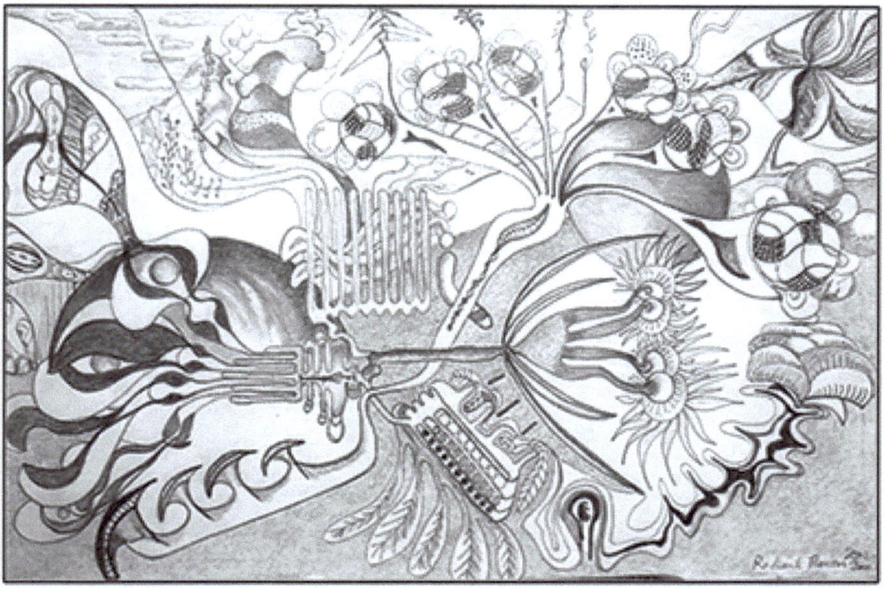

Radiant Flowers
Pencil
January 2011
41 x 28

Chapter 4
Development of the Doodle

At the beginning of October of 2010, I had already sunk to a very low level of depression, which was unfortunately to last until early 2011. Despite its gravity, I persisted in doodling, with only one occasion on which I used any other medium than pencil and paper. While art therapy can help, it does not always do so, and this is probably one very bad episode that was not clearly improved by doodling. But somehow my powers of concentration when doodling were not that eroded, and perhaps I became increasingly obsessed with my artwork. Idleness, where rest does not constitute a part of it, is anathema to me, so I would probably have been even worse if I had not continued to doodle. What proved quite extraordinary on reflection was the fact that I produced about 50 drawings, of which almost 20 are shown in the following pages. My partner, Jean, was equally surprised that such a lot had been produced in 3 months. Furthermore, the range of "subjects", "themes" or "patterns"—call them what you will, since all are abstract—was quite remarkable. [I might have apologised here for being very self-centred and a huge egotist if I had not been as astonished as my partner with the outcome in volume and detail. On reflection, the products often seems very alien to me—did I really do them?!] But from early days I had made quite a lot of large doodles, not just in 2010. Three of the more memorable images from earlier years follow.

D. N. Wheatley, *BipolART*,
DOI 10.1007/978-94-007-4872-9_4, © Springer Science+Business Media Dordrecht 2012

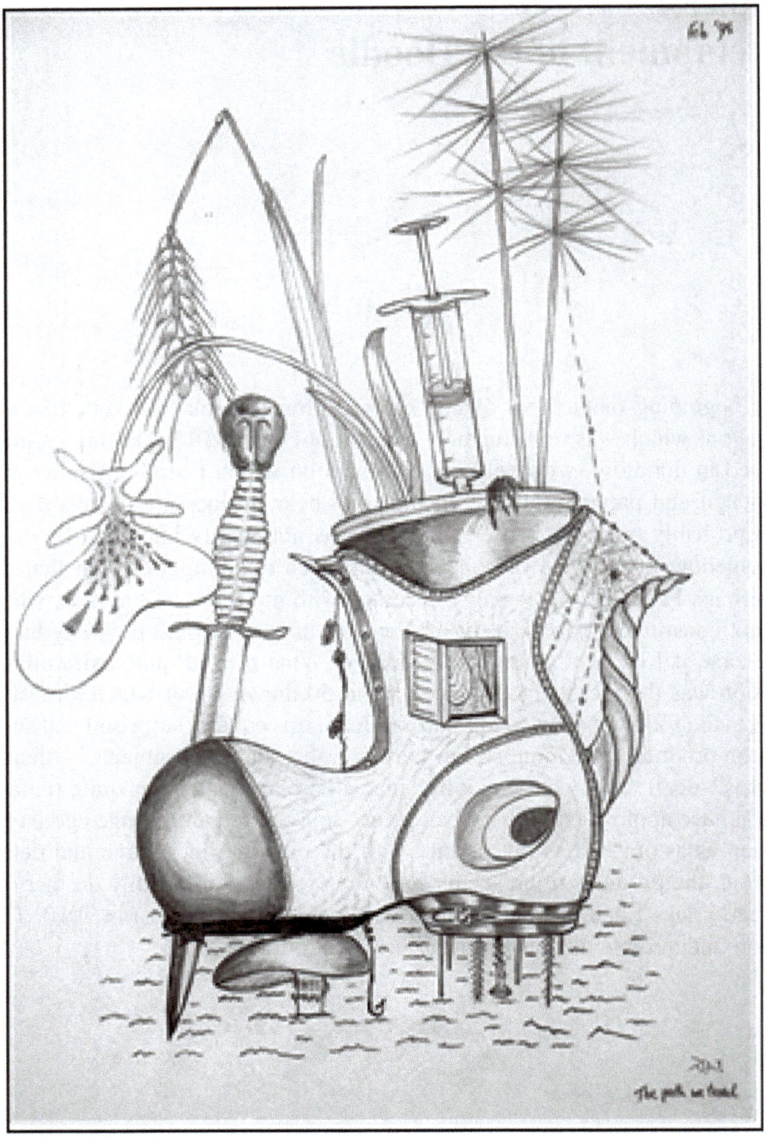

The paths we tread
February 1998
Pencil
20 x 34

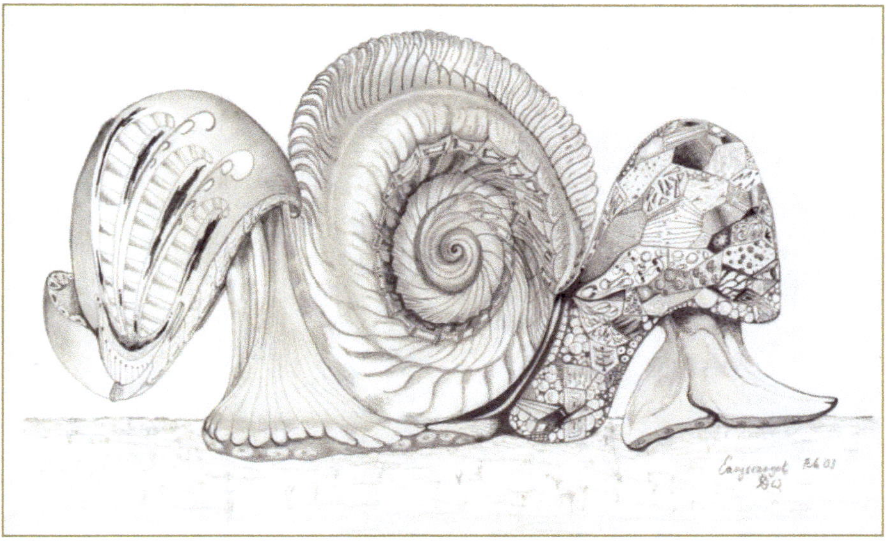

Easyscargot
February 2003
Pencil
36 x 24

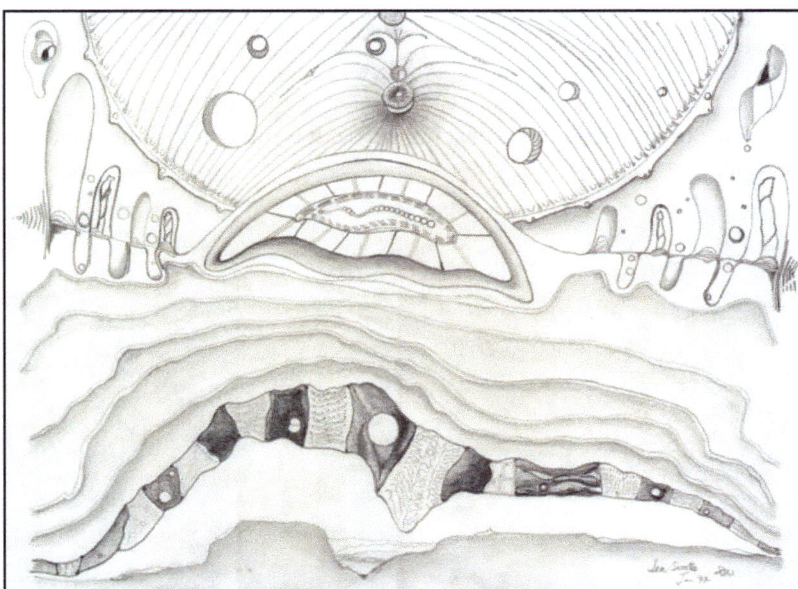

Sea scrolls
Pencil
January 1999
50 x 40

The biological background to these and the following are again very apparent, as in the nut-like (very embryonic) image that follows:

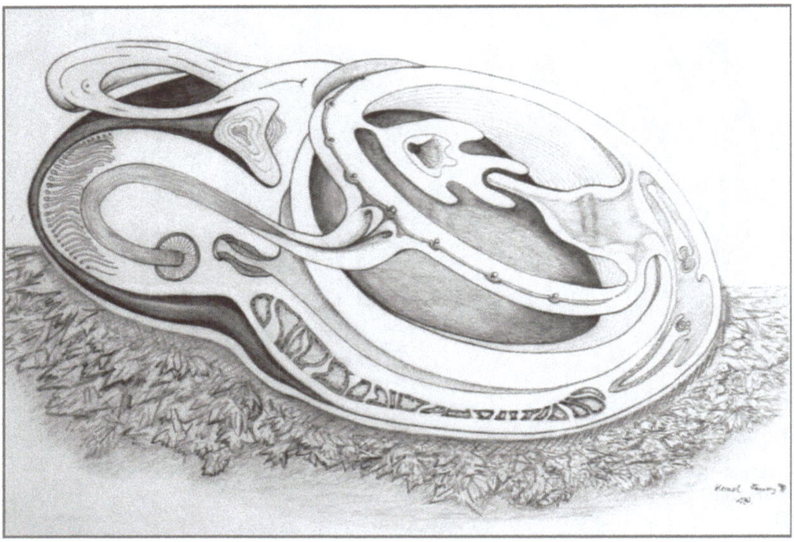

Kernel
January 1999
Pencil
32 x 23

There is much symbolism in the next image, but it is difficult to understand where it came from.

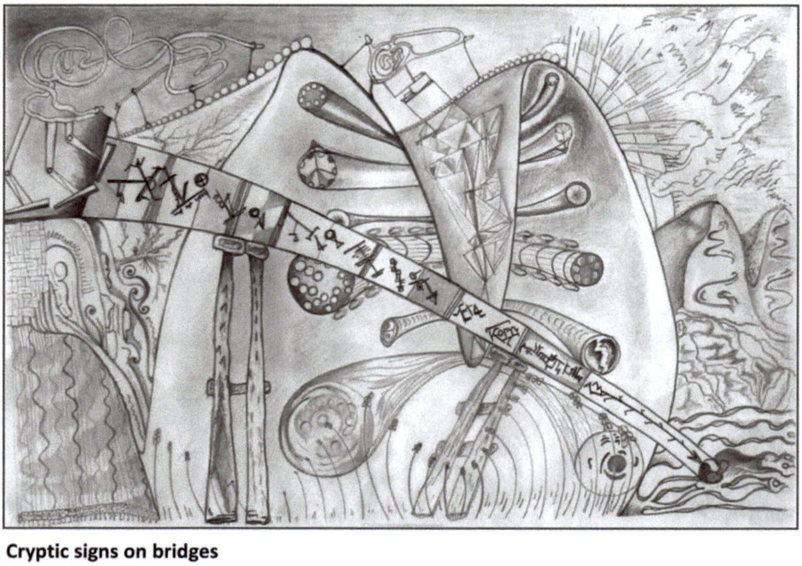

Cryptic signs on bridges
December 2004
Pencil
36 x24

The next three doodles are more in the style of the earlier forms, showing that this mode was still being used.

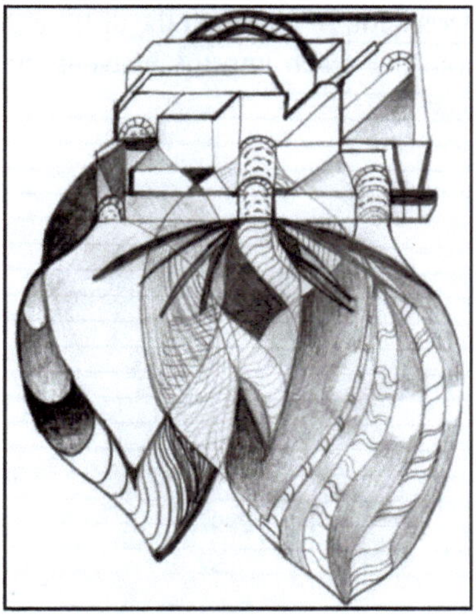

Pumping for air
December 2010
Pencil
15 x 18

The doodle above must have been a reminder many years later of human physiology practical classes held in Nottingham. Over the years, an increasing number of doodles developed into large works, with intricate detail, motifs and unusual features.

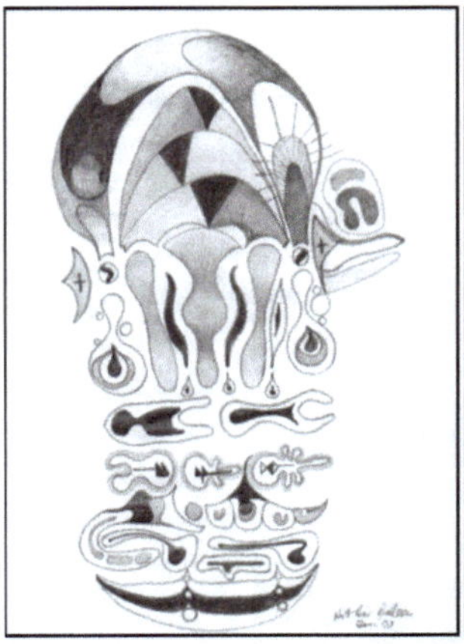

Hot air balloon
Pencil
January 2008
15 x 20

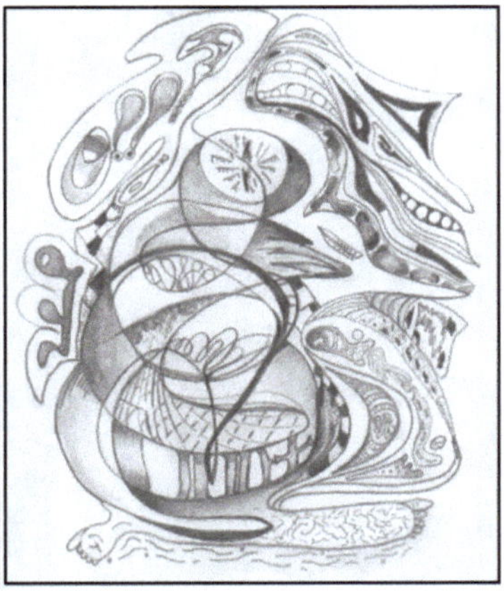

Planted feet
Pencil
January 2009
20 x 24

But now we come to an occasion where the doodle developed into a scene reminiscent of a Tower of Babel—an impression of a depiction by several other artists whose work was not in the forefront of my mind at the time, certainly not at the outsets, but probably in my subconscious—although the cliff on the right would suggest this structure that was not built to reach into the heavens, to be closer to God, as it is overshadowed in my case.

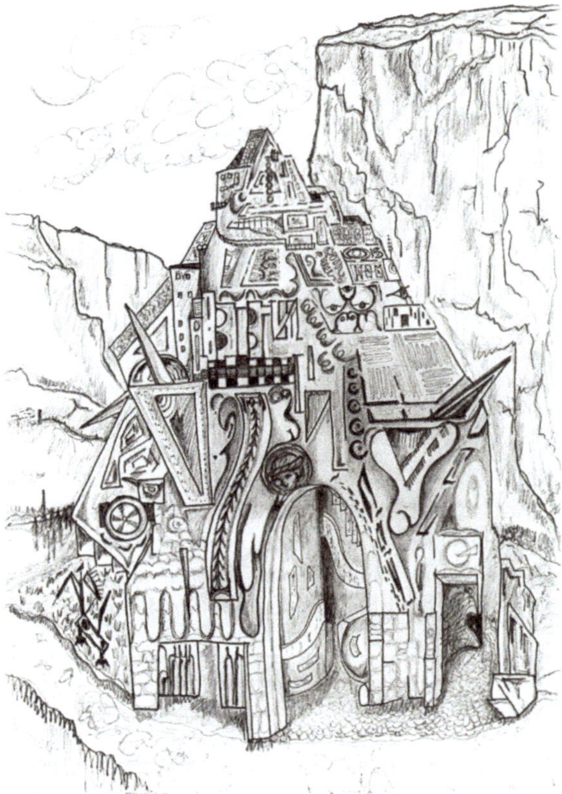

An old tower (of Babel?)

January 2006
Pencil, 14 x 22

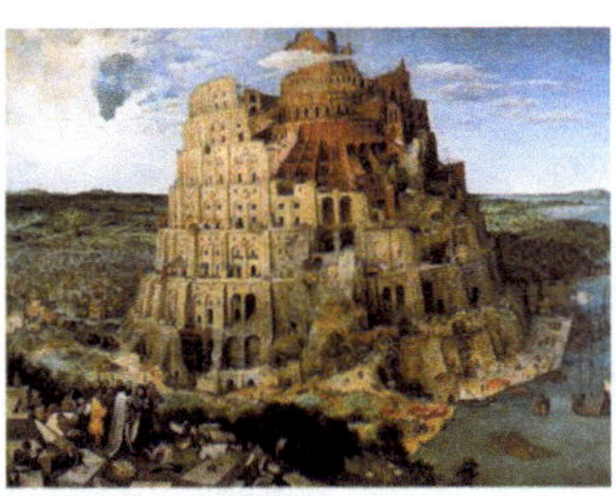

Breugel's Tower of Babel

It was a recurrent theme, as in a classical scene below, with castles in the mountains.

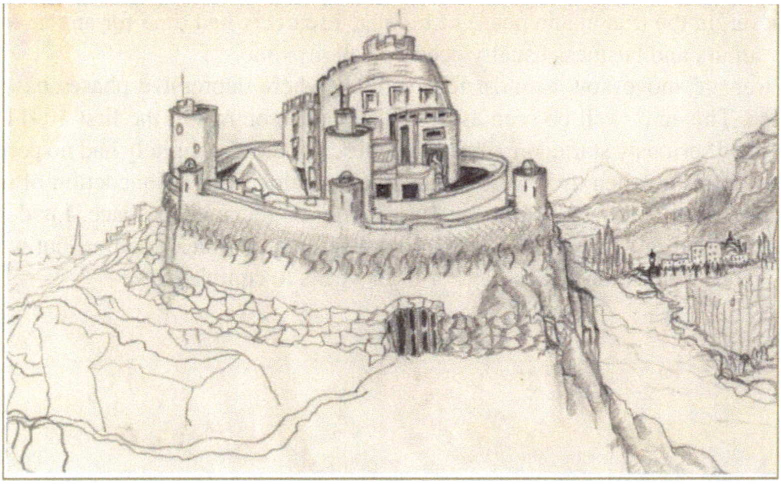

Old Fort
January 2007
Pencil
22 x 14

The tower or mountain theme (the following example having a rather phallic appearance) engendered a desire to create a colour picture on the same theme.

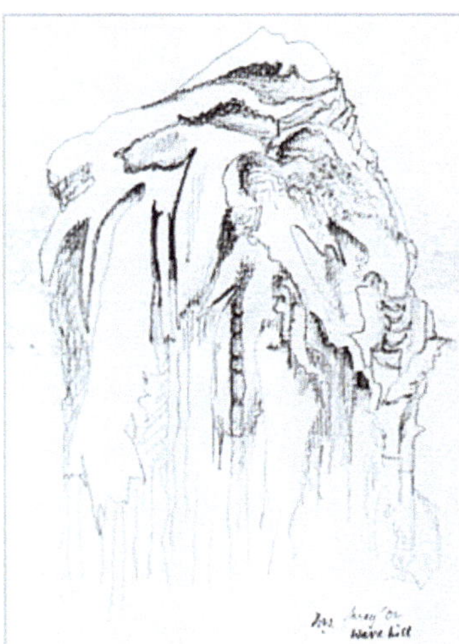

Wave Hill
May 2002
Pencil
12 x 18

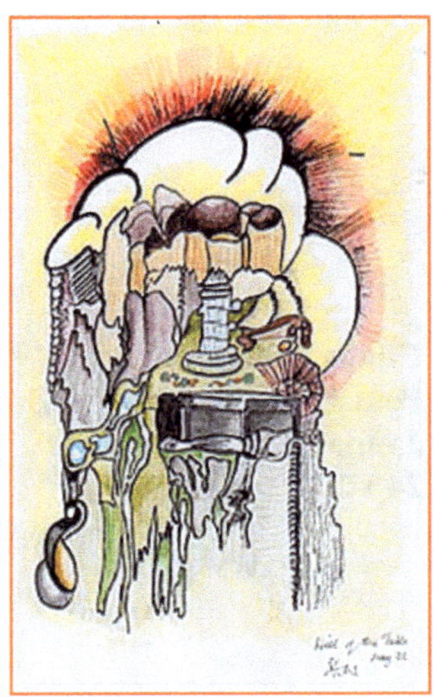

Hill of the table
May 2002
Pencil and crayon
10 x 18

Taking a doodle to new levels was usually done when I had recovered from the worst of the down phase and had more energy, driving me on to complete a grander work. However, in the true manic phase of bipolar, I scarcely had time for any artwork as other affairs and business usually occupied all my time.

I want to move now to most recent times where depressive phases have been intense. This may well be seen as of considerable contrast to the first 10–11 years after I had seriously started in 1998. With these doodles I definitely had no particular subject in mind when they were initiated, continuing to be a concoction of motifs, but now carefully confined in many cases within a rectangular space. I had indeed created a kind of genre of my own. Today I seldom do quick doodles, but work on these more stylized ones take days or even weeks to complete.

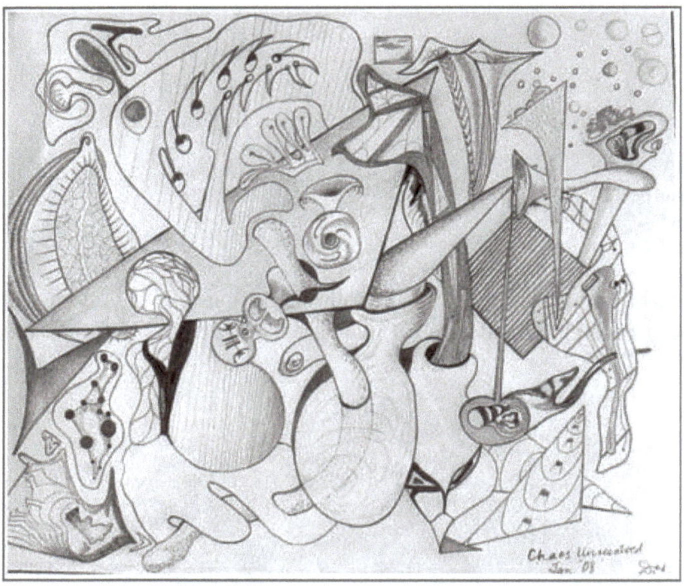

Chaos unresolved
Pencil
January 2008
24 x 20

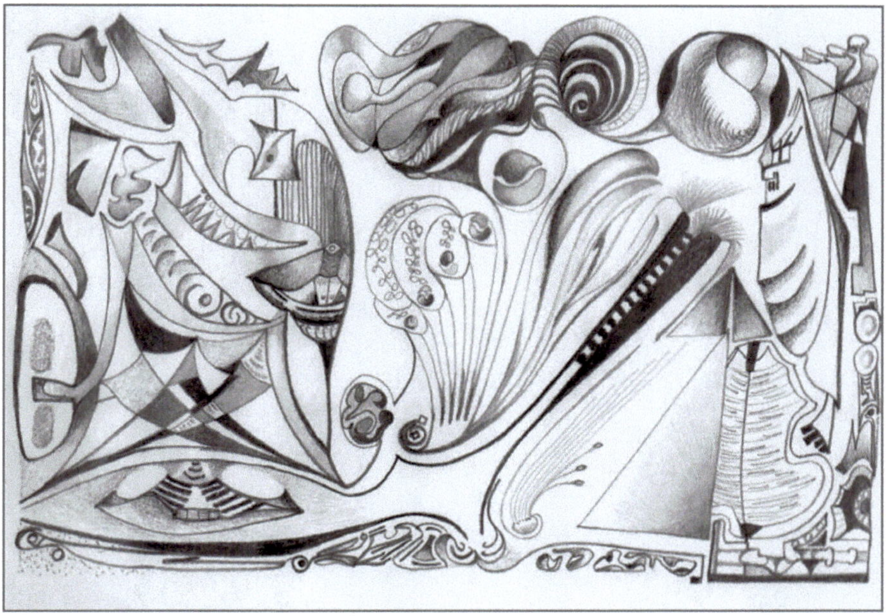

Untitled
Pencil
January 2011
24 x 18

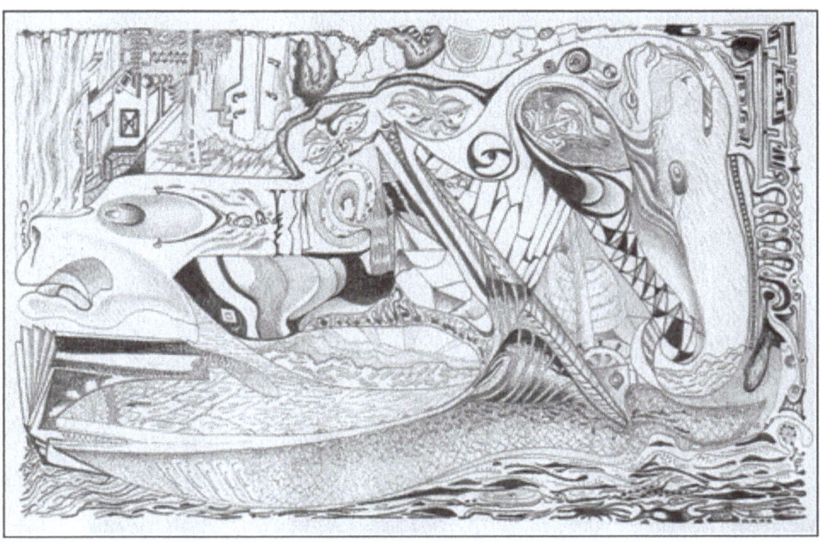

Leviathan
Pencil
February 2011
32 x 24

Chapter 5
A Biological Journey

There is no way of escaping the fact that I have had a long exposure throughout my career to familiar images seen in biology and medicine. My interest and inquisitiveness in all forms of life seem to have been present from about the age of four. At university, drawing specimens was a daily occurrence in anatomy, botany and other disciplines, and I did not find this taxing. In this chapter, the next room in the gallery, we are going through the biological and medical thema that have formed the basis of my life's work and clearly have had a dominant effect on the images—they cannot fail to reflect an absorbance in many aspects of nature. I have to reiterate that this speaks volumes of the close relationship between science and art. Much of classical art has been done by artists besotted with life-forms, especially the female body, by those in past centuries right up to today, many of whom were great artists—mainly men (fortunately not so now!).

The render will already have seen clear evidence of the biological basis of many of my doodles. These images often include the soft curvy lines of nature, which are in stark contrast to the other extreme where I have indulged in highly abstract concepts and geometrical forms (Chapter 10), although the former tend to be a mixture of the two, as you will see in subsequent chapters.

An early drawing of a reptile's skull (*Varanus*) is seen first in this chapter, one of many hundreds of similar drawings done in my undergraduate days over 50 years ago. The following picture reiterates this same form, but I was totally unaware I was doing it in 2001; in fact these drawings were done 53 years apart. Soon after drawing this, a doodle on page 44 began that took the form of a dragon (why are dragons usually depicted as reptiles?), and this turned into a most elaborate painting in acrylics called "fantasy birds" page 45. The doodle was done during deep depression, but the painting was completed during a manic period some 4 months later. It is obvious that there are strong underlying themes involved here that range from the natural to the fantastic. I scarcely referred to books on birds to paint these images, as explained in the Prologue. Somehow they just seemed to be there in my mind, and that is as spooky to me as it might seem to you. I attributed this to something of an eidetic memory (which no longer seems to work so well), but has somehow allowed me to retain most of the images I have stored away in my mind (brain) from a much earlier age when I would totally immerse myself in encyclopedias, manuals and reference books of all

D.N. Wheatley, *BipolART*,
DOI 10.1007/978-94-007-4872-9_5,

kinds, as well as observing the real things. What is equally odd to me as an amateur musician is that my earlier eidetic memory failed me completely in memorising music; I have to have the music before me, although I took compensation in being a competent sight-reader.

Later my focus became much more involved with sub-microscopic aspects of life than gross anatomy, since I was researching the ultrastructure of minute biological structures in cells soon after the electron microscope became standard in a well-equipped biomedical department. Some of the images that follow are indeed impressions of cellular and subcellular life-forms.

While animals and other living creatures have always been a fascination, I have often merges real life and abstract forms of both plants and animals; some of the later pictures in this "gallery" illustrate this admixture.

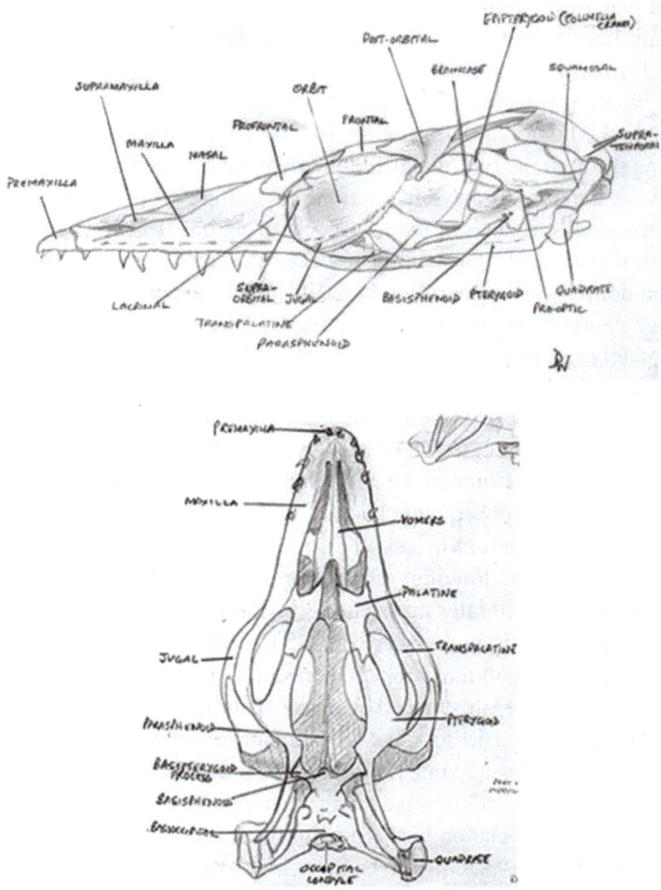

Varanus
Pencil
1959
14 x 8 (both)

The skull motif is so obvious in this next and other pictures done in the present period (1998–2011). This one below was done 42 years after the ones on the previous page.

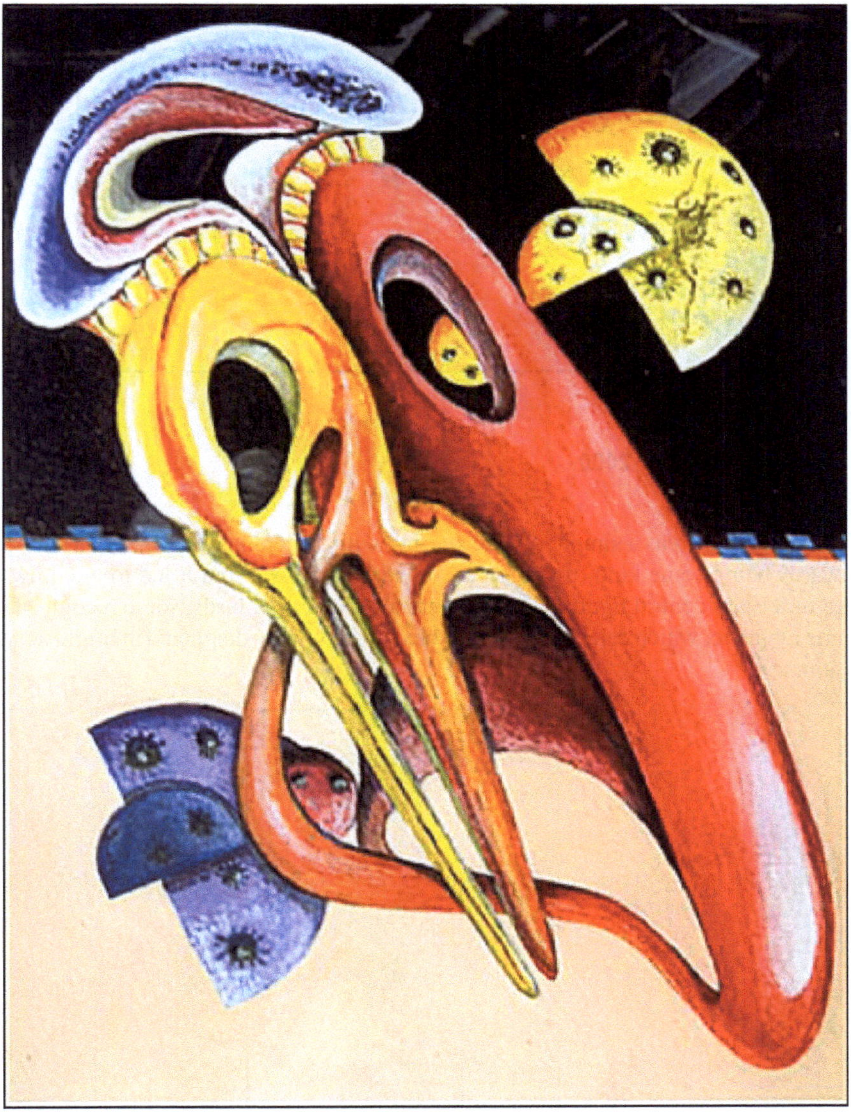

Moons and Skulls
Acrylics
December 2001
33 x 23

In the picture below, the image seems to be that of a pelvic girdle in part of a skeleton, but seems to incorporate some rather obvious fleshy tissues!

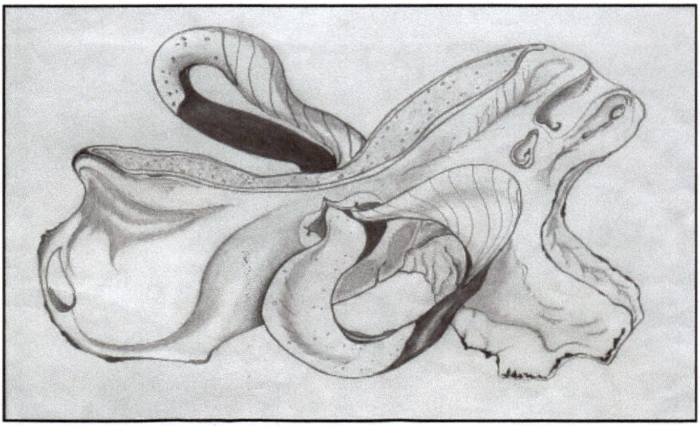

Bony Girdle
Pencil
December 2000
35 x 25

This next image was a simple doodle starting with sweeping curves—it was moving towards being some kind of dragon as already mentioned, but it led to a redrawing as a bird (dark central figure), and then into a collection of birds, some recognisable, some fantastic, which can be seen on the next page, vividly displayed in bright acrylic colours.

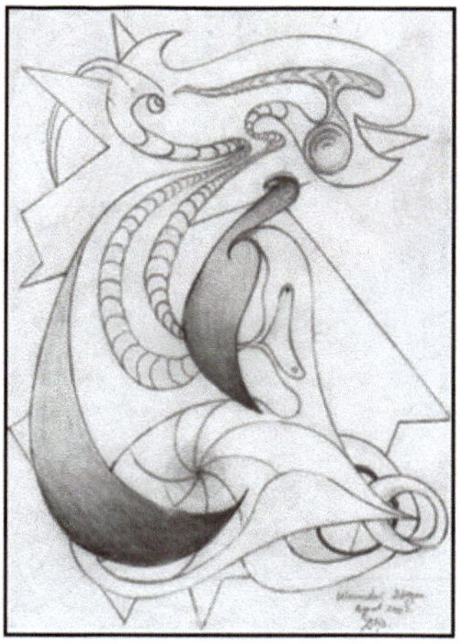

Wounded Dragon
Pencil
April 2002
30 x 20

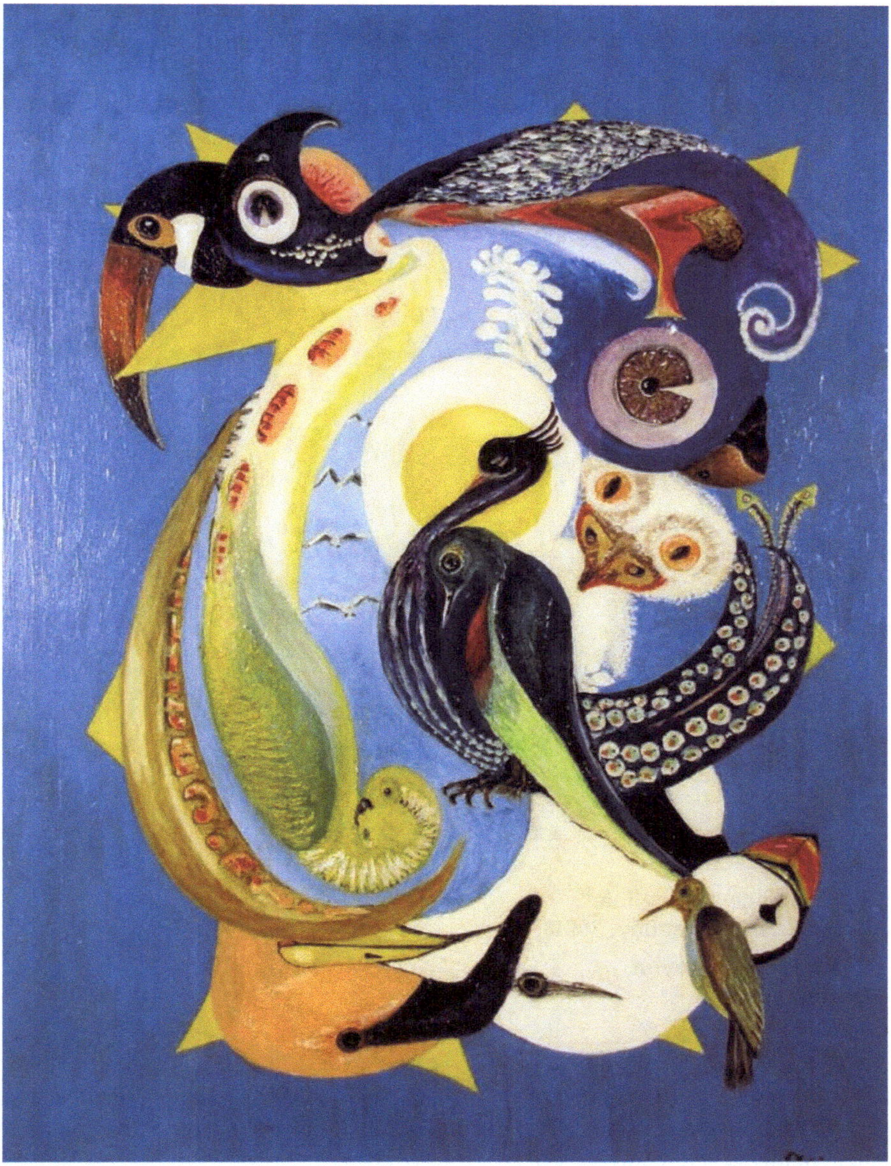

Fantasy Birds
Acrylics
April 2002
40 x 30

A melancholy bird? Oh! Idle thought!
In Nature there is nothing melancholy.
(Coleridge-Taylor: *The Nightingale*)

Biological motifs have been drawn together deliberately in the following doodle, which started as a bit of brain just right of centre. At the time, I was co-authoring a book entitled *About Life* with Dr. Paul Agutter, also published by Springer. The doodle later became increasingly elaborate as I moved out of depression and took on even more intricacy when it was seen as a potential Frontispiece for the book. Most of the structures depicted in it are at the cellular or subcellular level, such as blood cells coursing along a vein at the bottom. This was also the start of doing most doodles "within a definite frame".

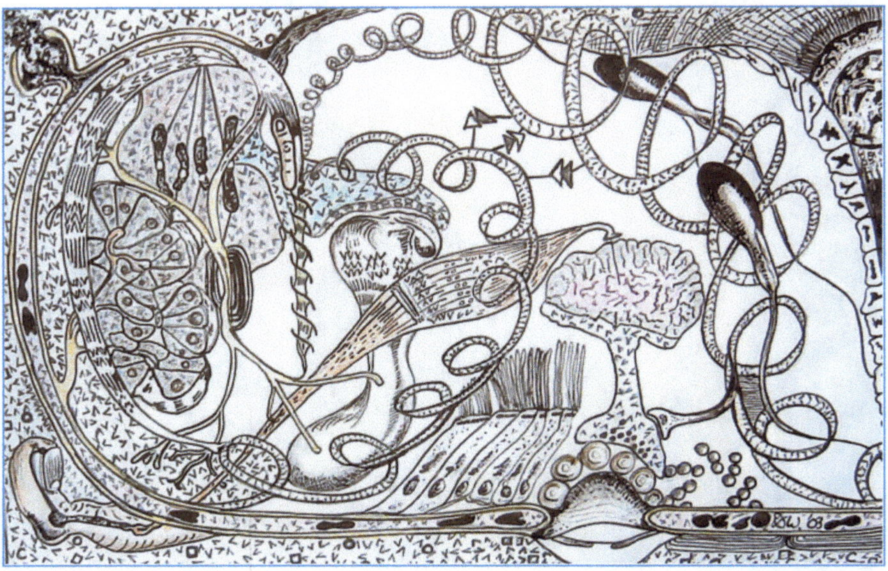

Frontispiece "About Life"
(Agutter and Wheatley, 2008)

Black ink and crayon
December 2006
21 x 14

The two watercolour paintings below bear, intentionally, a vague resemblance to single and double-stranded DNA molecules, the code of life, but why I depicted them in this way remains a mystery.

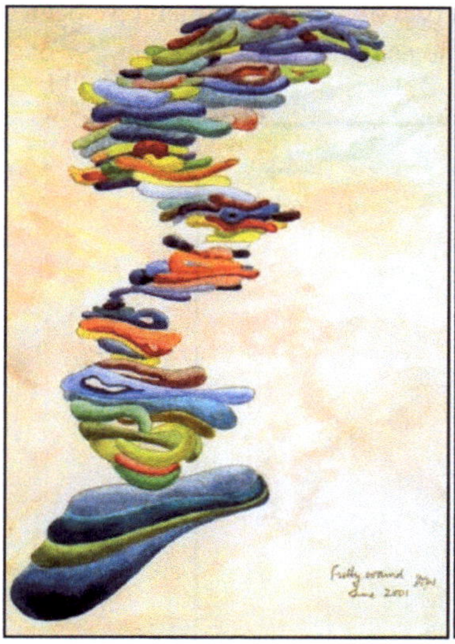

Fully Wound
Watercolour
July 2001
25 x 18

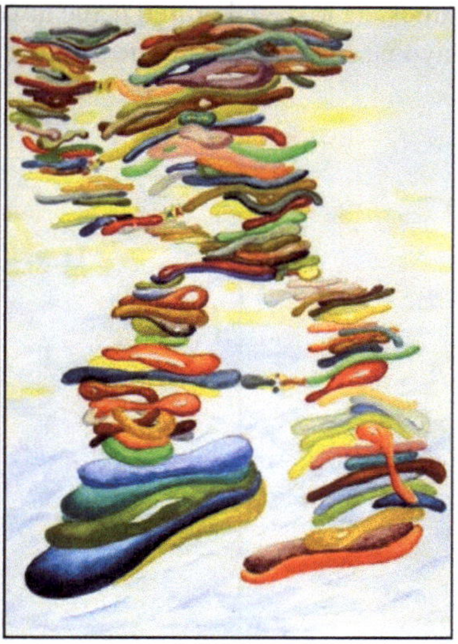

Doubly Wound
Watercolour
July 2001
33 x 23

The small doodle below had almost the same idea at the chromosome level with its banding, showing a kernel (nucleus) seemingly directing the development of fingers.

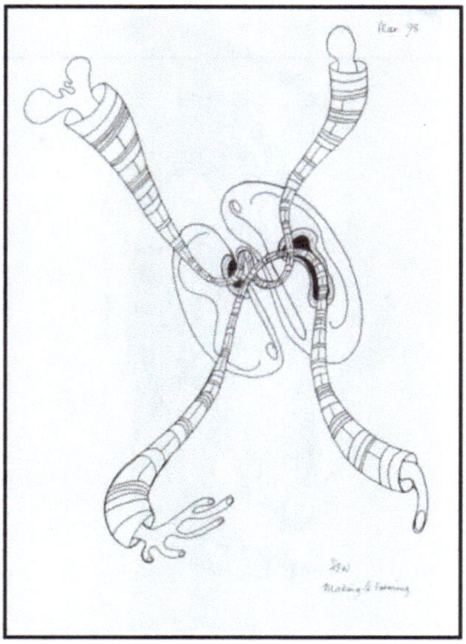

Making and Forming
Pencil
March 1998
16 x 12

Pipes, tubes, hearts are featured in the next two small doodles that have been coloured with crayons, drawn at much the same time as bony girdle image a few pages back.

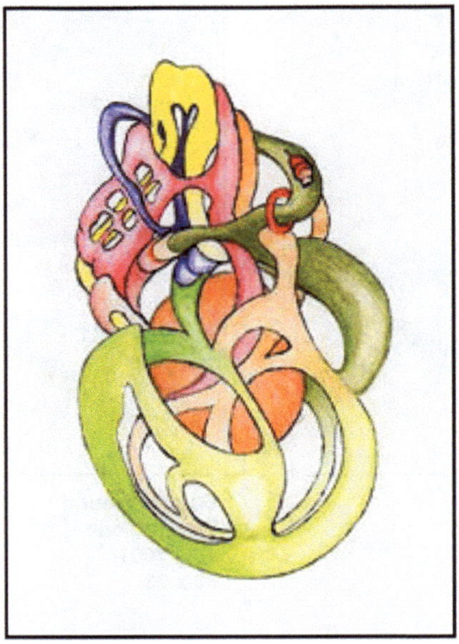

Circulation
Pencil and crayon
June 2001
12 x 8

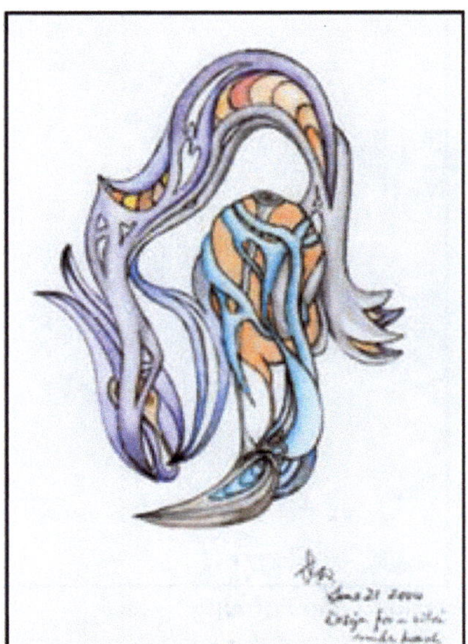

Design for a silver brooch
Pencil and crayon
June 2001
12 x 8

Joinging the animal and vegetal worlds has been tried on anumber of occasions, with the picture below called Shellflower being an example. It incorporates more than just a shell-like structures, as can be seen particuarly at its underside, but more fleshy parts. And embedded within the shell is an orange flower. There is also a blue-purple spiral structure near the flower, which might be quite inanimate; this is a recurrent motif in my work. The picture was done in 2004, and cannot be other than closely related to the blue spiral drawing seen on page 76, which had been completed in 2001. Helical structures, among them shells, feature prominently in nature, both at the macroscopic and microscopic levels, right down to the macromolecular basis of life itself in the molecule of DNA. Clearly it is a form that is constantly in my mind and will be found throughout many of the other pictures in this book.

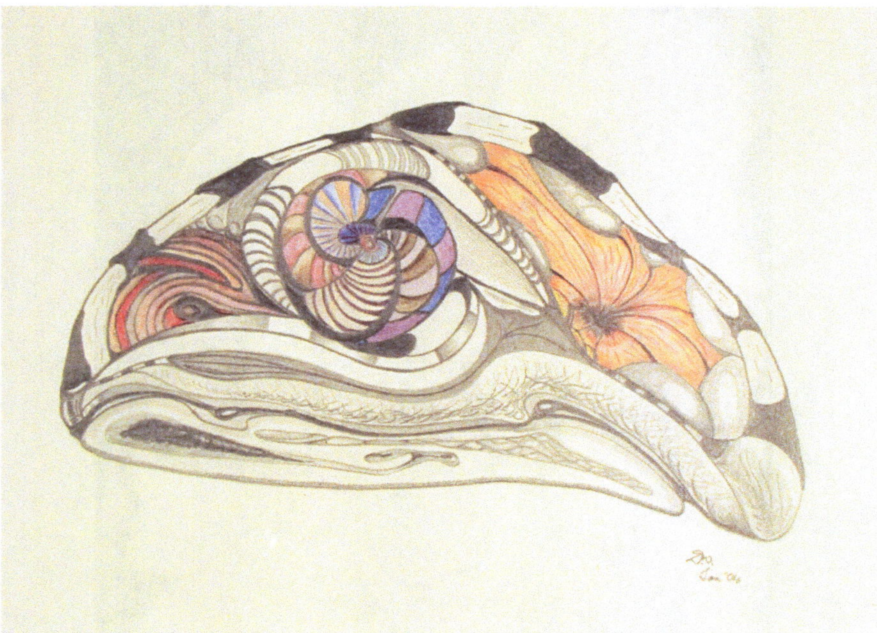

Shellflower
Pencil and Crayon
January 2004
36 x 27

Tell us, pray, what devil
This melancholy is, which can transform
Men into monsters.
(John Ford: *The Lady's Trial*)

The exercise below was one of direct drawing and painting in thick acrylics of a stem of orchids. As one of the early paintings of the years being covered, this became an obsession, the objective being to make the petals as fleshy as in real life as possible, which was partially successful. I believe my first long session in 1998 of doodling had revived in me an interest in doing some more conventional art. The drawing of orchids took only a short time, but the painting took ages to get right, which was done after I had recovered following its start at the end of 1999.

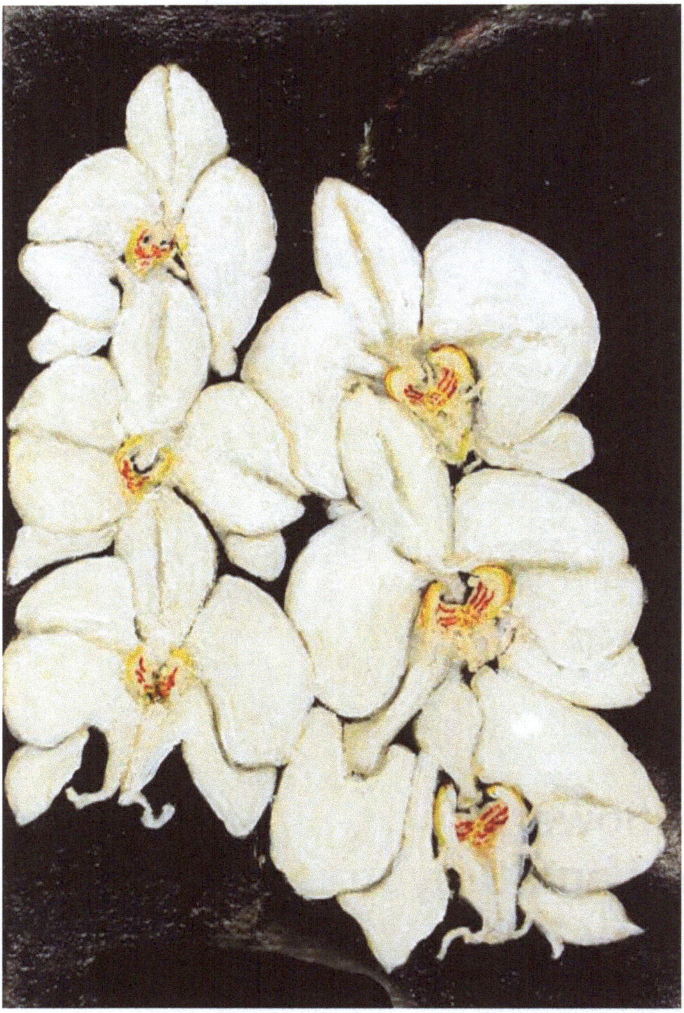

Orchids
Acrylics
December 1999
20 x 12

The next picture done when falling into a depression in 2010 is a faithful sketch of a very old tree devoid of leaves seen in Manchester.

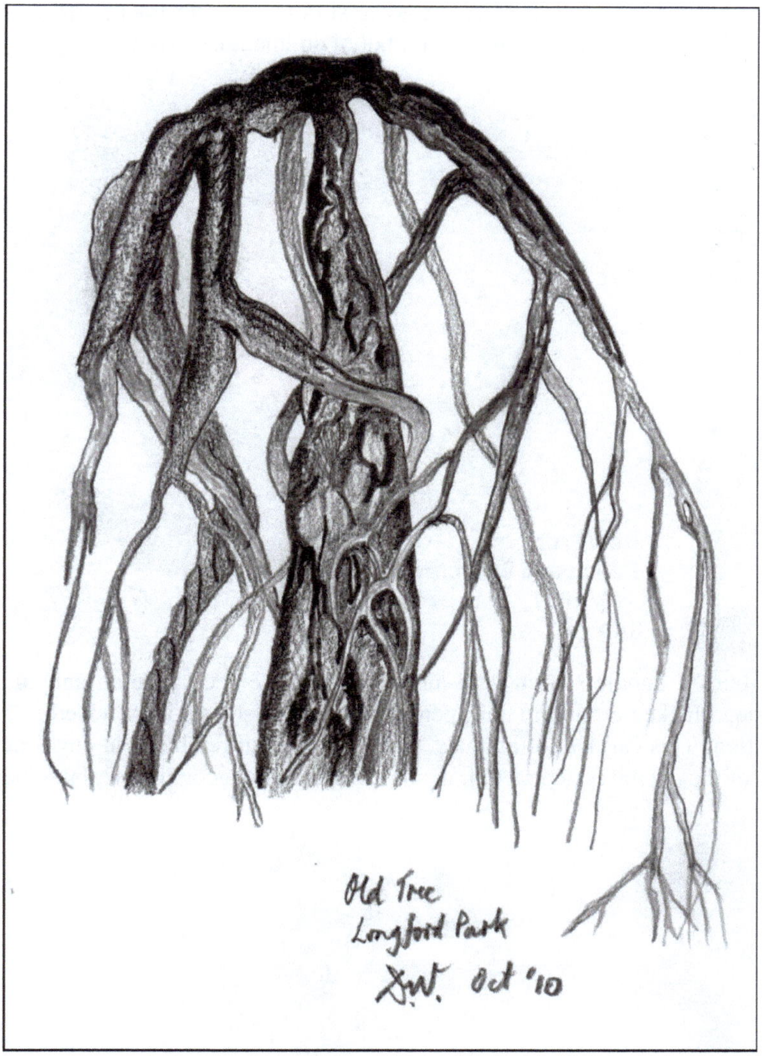

Old Tree
Longford Park (Manchester)
Pencil
12 x 16

But from obvious reality, it is quite easy to shift to more abstract portrayal of life-forms. The following picture is of fruit, but of an imaginary kind.

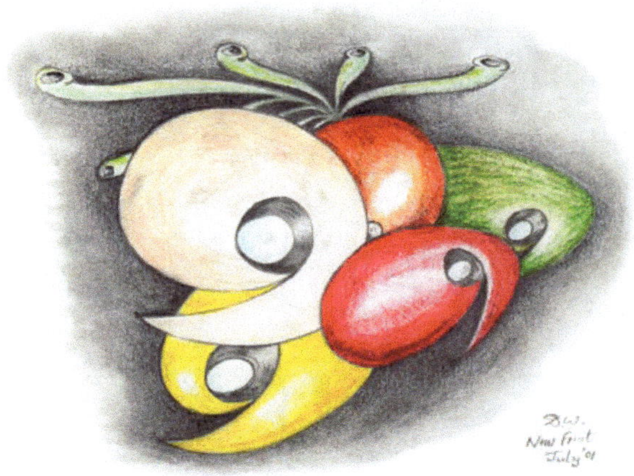

New Fruit
Pencil and wax crayon
July 2001
14 x 16

Sometimes a doodle started with an outline of an object, here an animal, which was then blocked around in dark pencil while other shapes were added to create a collection. This carnival of animals was done without reference at any time to the shape of the creatures depicted in it, some being quite recognizable, but others not.

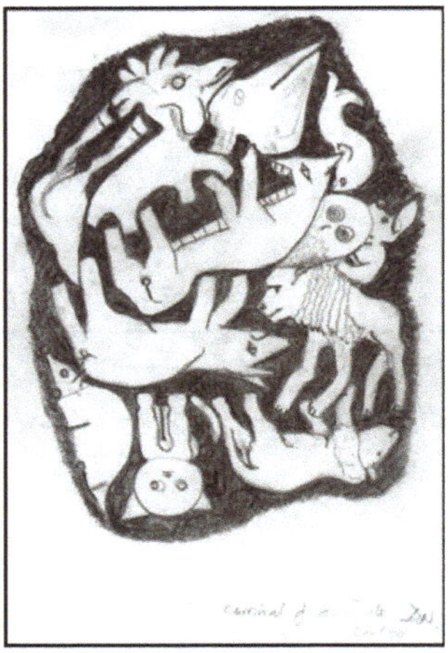

Carnival of animals
Pencil
December 2004,
16 x 22

But plants seaweed and shells have all clearly been represented as in the next doodle, although I am an animal man more than a botanical person.

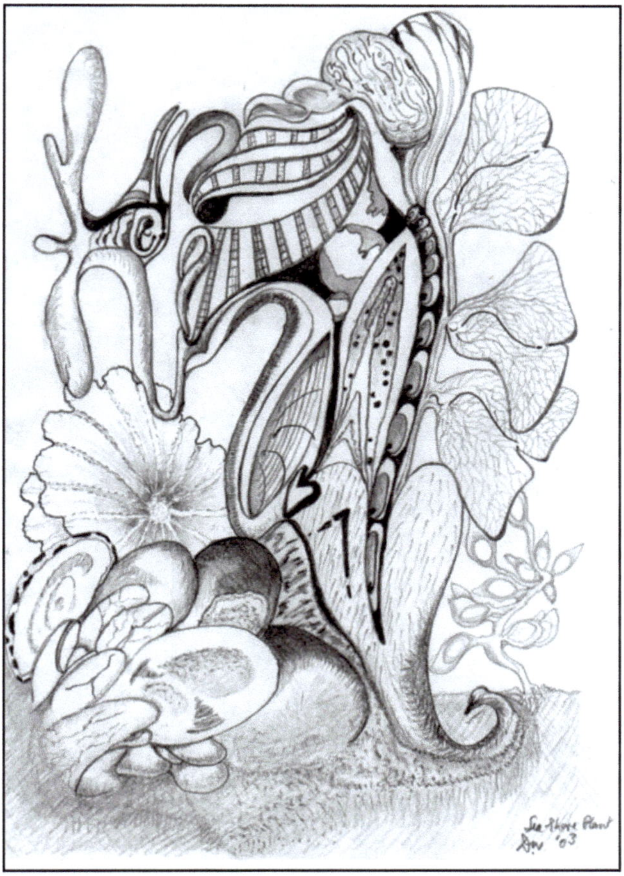

Seashore plant
Pencil
December 2003
16 x 29

And such a want-wit sadness makes me,
That I have so much ado to know myself.
(Shakespeare: *The Merchant of Venice*)

Chapter 6
Reality—Drawings from Life

Human kind cannot very much bear reality.
(Thomas Stearns Eliot: *Burnt Norton*)

My first picture in this chapter is a bit on an anomaly, an anachronism with regard to the period being covered (1998–2011). Unlike the doodle discovered from student days in chapter 2 (Writer's World, page 10), the drawing here is one of reality, an accurate representation of a Christmas rose, done during the start of a depression in November 1989. It was not found until clearing out a draw that I used to keep some of my old pencils, paints and other paraphernalia associated with art. I do remember one thing about it, which was that my wife at that time suggested I do some artwork as I had done many years before in America. The difference here from any other picture is that I wrote my feelings in the top left-hand corner, something I have not done since, which in some ways is a pity because there would also have been words conveying some of my feelings when it was being drawn. However, a picture of this kind resembling an actual object is unlikely to convey much emotion! It is a sizable pencil drawing on an A3 sheet of paper.

Accurate representation is an attempt to capture the actual nature of a subject, like a "still life". Some feeling can be put into it in terms of its accuracy, colour and context, but not when it is little more than a picture that comes close to a photograph reproduction. However, reality is life as you see it, and it may differ considerably from what others see. With different mind-sets, reality as conventionally understood (by consensus) can be quite dramatically changed from this "reality"—I show one example where a familiar building to all in the locality is followed by another ("Dacha") that is an imaginary building of the same type. But if some artwork portrays something which is easily recognizable to others, as is the case with the lodge house, then there is little question about what it is and in this case where it is. A neighbour shown these pictures or the one entitled "The farm enface" would instantly recognize both of them.

D. N. Wheatley, *BipolART*,
DOI 10.1007/978-94-007-4872-9_6, © Springer Science+Business Media Dordrecht 2012

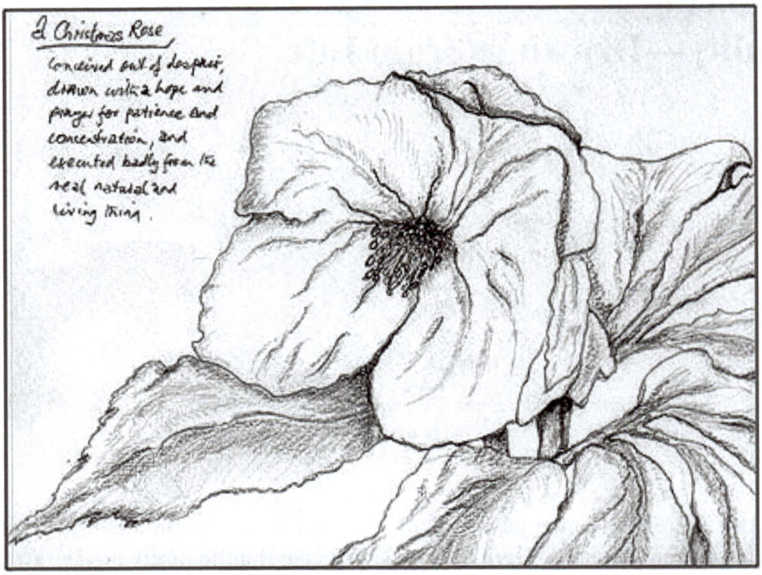

A Christmas Rose
Pencil
November 1989
27 x 24

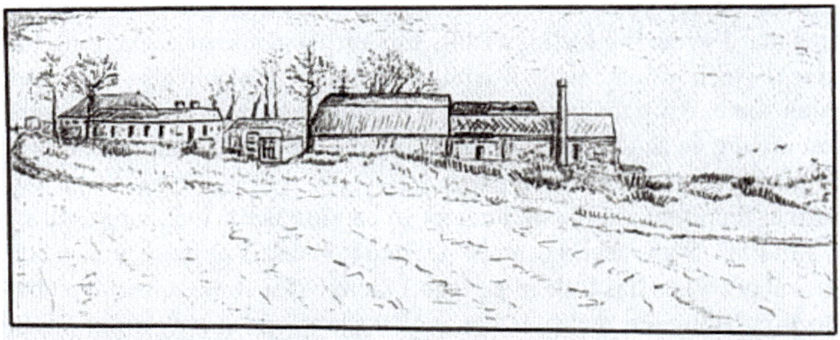

The farm enface
Indian Ink
January 2006
28 x 14

Equally, the next picture is a true likeness of the South Lodge of the Viscount of Kintore's seat called "Keithhall", which is literally just down the road from my house. It is so unusual in design that no one for miles around would mistake this for anything else, as the photograph taken after the drawing attests. The sketch on the right of the photograph gives a slightly different view.

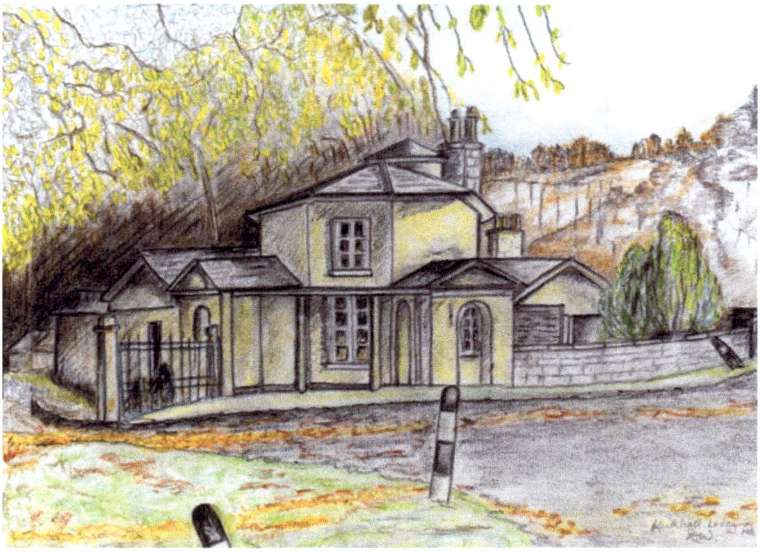

South Lodge, Keithhall
Pencil and crayon
February 2006
32 x 20

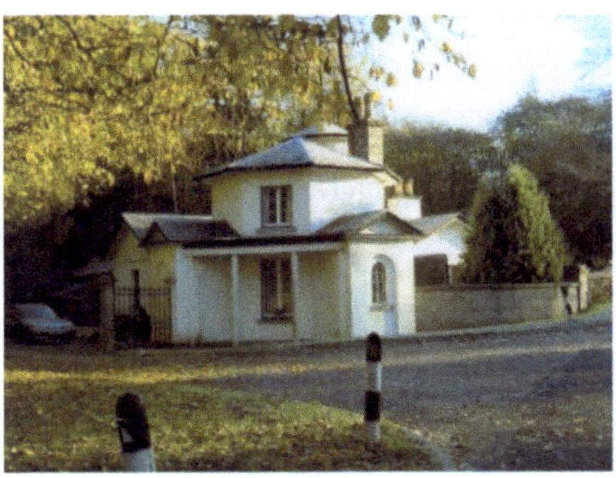

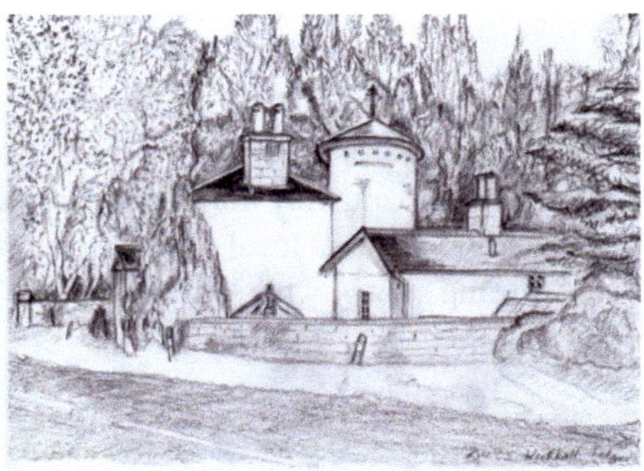

Pencil, February 2006, 32 x 20

But I went on to imagine something different. This is not a recognizable depiction of the same lodge house nearby; however, if you were to see the two pictures above after seeing this drawing, you would not mistake the resemblance. My thoughts at the time had probably drifted from a formal lodge house to a dacha out in the wilds of Russia!

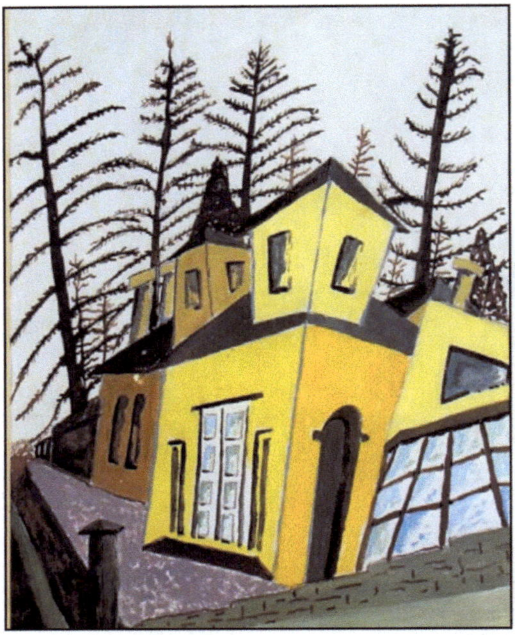

"Dacha"
Watercolour
March 2006
22 x 32

Below the situation is different. Sunset over a nearby mountain is something like this, only comparatively much more resplendent. The drawing is not accurate, but is close enough for any local inhabitant to recognize this well known "monument". I was learning slowly what "artistic license" meant!

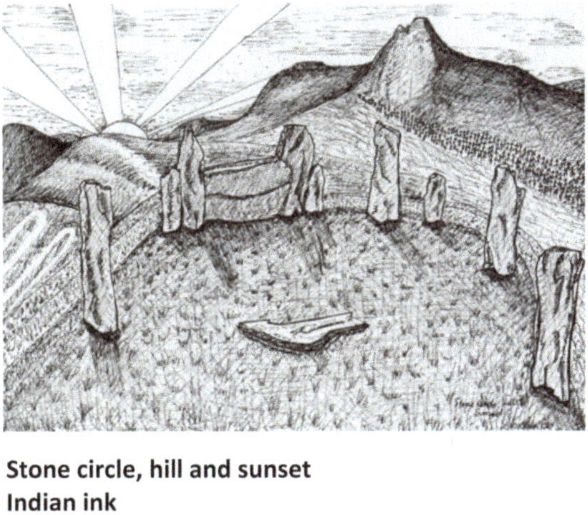

Stone circle, hill and sunset
Indian ink
January 2008
30 x 21

I could sit drawing the same mountain (Bennachie) time and again. But as time passes, so your view keeps changing—*panta rei, ouden menei* (everything flows, nothing remains still)—here three times.

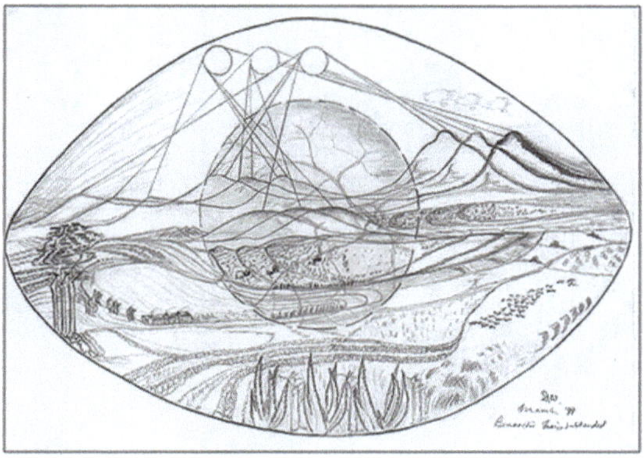

Bennachie thrice subtended
Pencil
March 1998
40 x 30

The eye is seeing the view above, but the actual eye that is beholding the scene simply cannot be included—it is a physical impossibility. For those who think about this deeply I recommend the interesting book by Douglas Harding *On having no head.*

Reality was something I strongly had in mind in March 2004 when I had recovered enough from a long Winter depression to be dragged away by my wife and two friends for a 2-week holiday in Madeira. It's an odd island, lashed the day we got there by incredible winds and rain, so much so that the rivulets ran with orange-red watery mud, with all the iron ore in it, coming in torrents off the near 45° mountain slopes. The drawings on the island were mostly in pencil, but I did resort to watercolour for the sea, flowers and trees.

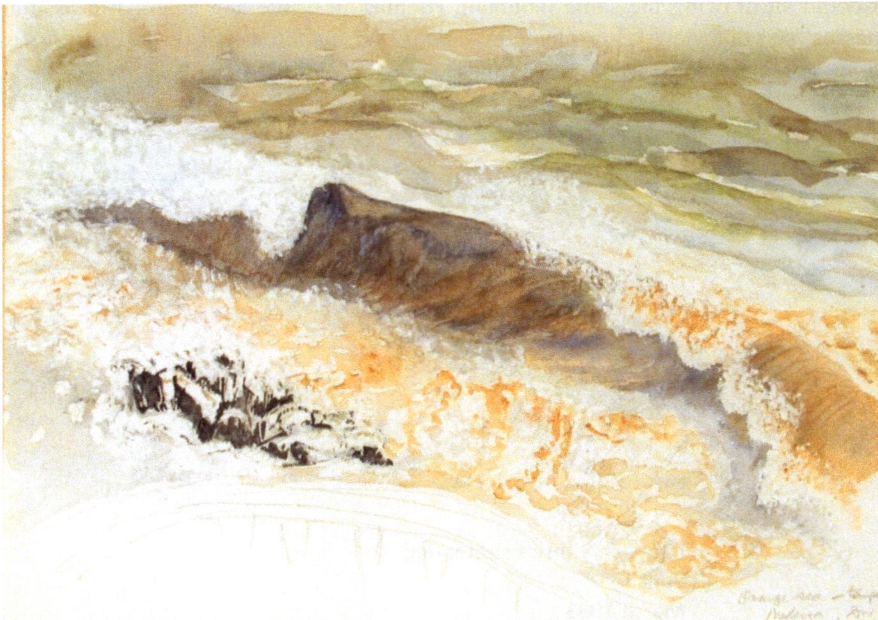

Orange sea – tempest, Madeira
Watercolour
March 2001
32 x 22

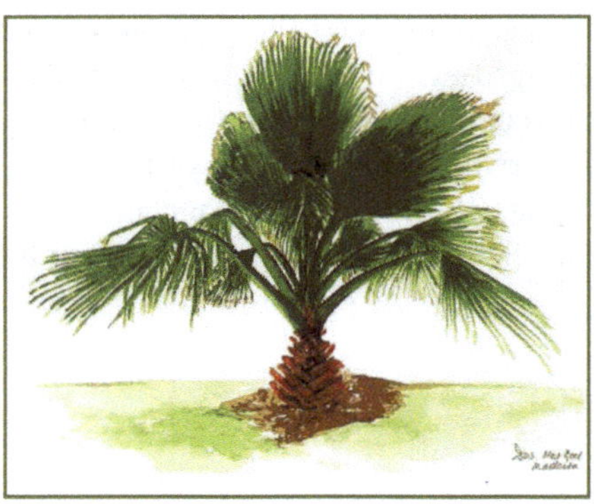

Palm tree, Madeira

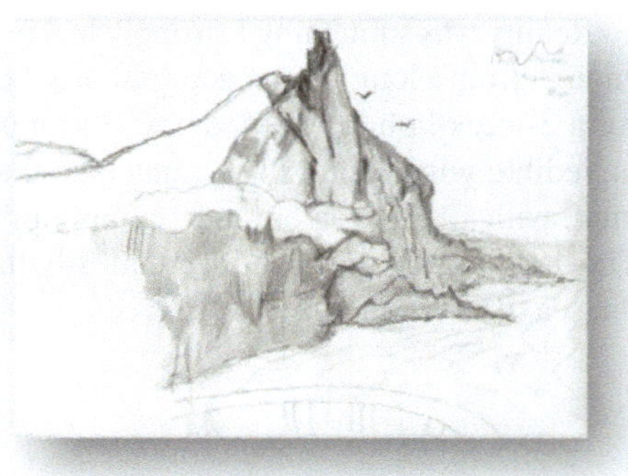

St Laurence point, Madeira

I had a similar experience about 4–5 years later at the same time of the year after a deep depression. My new partner and I were trying to relax after the worst of my trough by going to another island, this time Holy Island (Lindisfarne), off the Northumbrian coast in England. Driving towards it one day, I asked Jean to stop by a farm-gate to sketch the island from a distance and then paint it later. What was a

10–15 minutes sketch later became transformed into a sizeable painting. By coincidence, a storm had passed over the island and was disappearing off to the South, but the effect was quite magical. To have captured it has since given some pleasure, although many of my paintings can be painful in reflection.

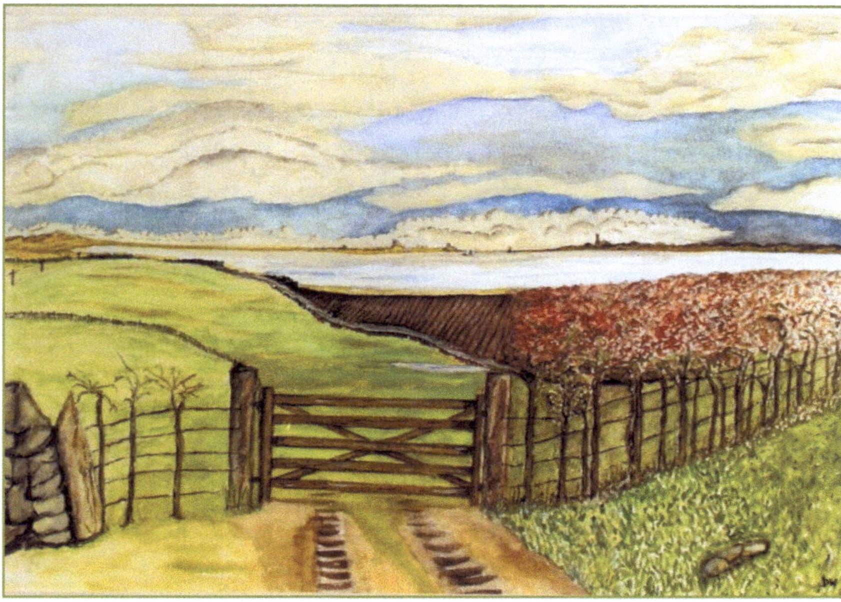

Holy Island - Lindisfarne
Watercolour
February 2005
42 x 31

One of my latest sketches (of several) was done at Macchu Picchu, but of the village and not the usual scenic view at the top of the peak nearby. We had 3 hours to wait for a train back to Obuntitomba. Two similar sketches were done from the bank of the river, one looking upstream and the other downstream. It took about 90 minutes to complete this one. We were on vacation in Peru, and I was in a good mood, and the pencil just seemed to take over!

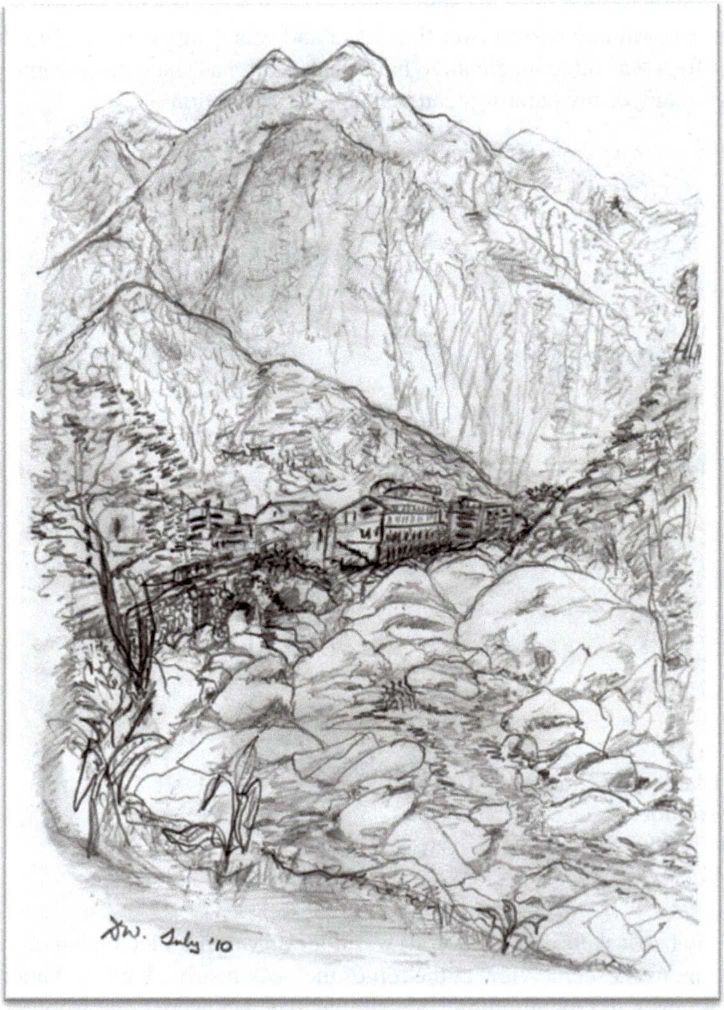

Macchu Picchu village
Pencil
July 2010
22 x 32

Sometimes I do portraits and life-drawings, but not many of them turn out to be a reasonable likeness of the subject. I was particularly pleased with the ones below of Una (nude on left) and Daniella (on right). The portrait below these two on the left was really pleasing—a very good likeness of the sitter (a biker called Mike). These three sketches were done on Saturday mornings at The Scarab Club—an art club—in Detroit, and I was the only foreign member. It was just two blocks from Wayne State Medical School where I had been working. Bottom right is Douglas, an old friend whom I sketched shortly before he died. Only afterwards seeing a photograph of him did I appreciate how much I had caught his wry smile; before that, I was not happy with it.

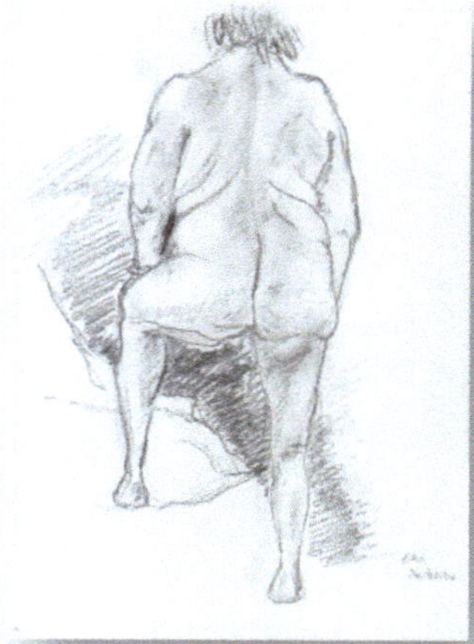

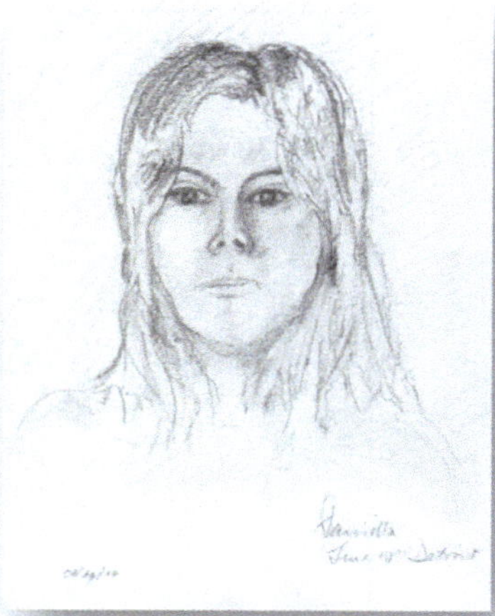

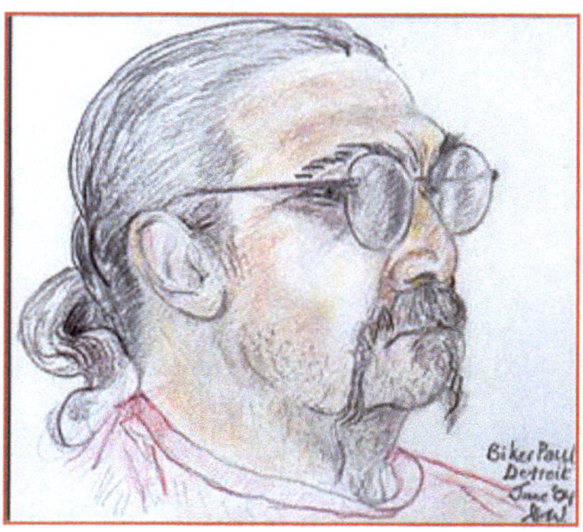

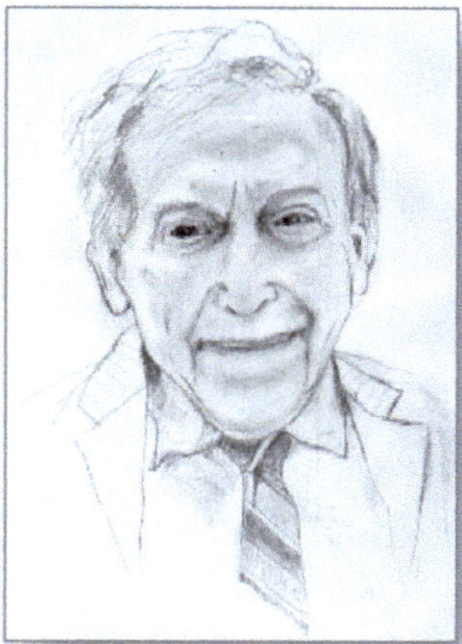

What we see is not what we draw; it's only our impression or interpretation of it at that time. The state of the mind will usually determine how it wants to interpret something. van Gogh painted many canvasses in the 4–5 months before his death. One of them shown below is an idyllic peaceful cherry orchard and the next depicts cypress trees on a hillside—they were drawn only a month or two apart, and their completely different styles must reveal changes from serenity to deep anguish in van Gogh's mind. This brings home the point that art can reveal the inner state of the mind. Equally remarkably, these two pictures were within a meter of each other when I last saw them in the National Gallery of Scotland.

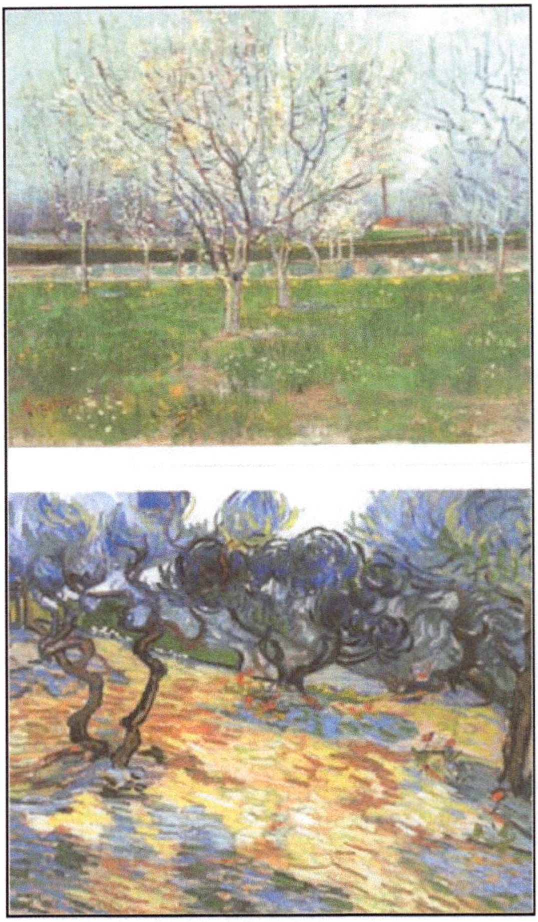

Two late van Gogh's Showing highly contrasting approaches used during the last few months of his life.

Chapter 7
A Short Musical Interlude

The great geniuses suffer and must suffer, but they need not complain;
they have known intoxication unknown to the rest of us and,
if they wept tears of sadness, they have poured tears of ineffable joy.
That in itself is a heaven for which one never pays what it is worth.
(Charles Gounod: Composer)

Music has always been not only very important to me, both as a listener and a player, but is an integral part of my life. In times of deep depression, listening to particular pieces of music can have a very soothing effect, but concentrating aurally has to be built up over time because often a "loved" piece can be emotionally upsetting and gets switched off very quickly. Sometimes the attention span is too short and the music in not appreciated. Background music is a no-no for me during depression, but I wonder if it is important for others. I am more in need of quiet than anything else.

One of the early and enduring manifestations of severe depression is the inability to play music. Very little seems to "come naturally"; it is all hard work and the sound you get out of instruments is quite awful. The lack of concentration and dexterity (motor coordination) can be devastating, and that is why the cello and piano get ignored throughout most of depression. This is a great disappointment because I derive much pleasure from playing and performing in a number of orchestras both at home and abroad. I have played in them on a couple of occasions when depressed because I had been utterly committed to doing so, and surprisingly was complimented by a couple of friends who knew I was suffering, but said that I managed very well. They would not have known just how much this took out of me, with utter exhaustion for a couple of days.

When well on the way to recovering from depression, one is quite aghast at the speed with which satisfactory performance is regained, and how easy it suddenly seems. Listening to long pieces of music starts to become a pleasure again. An all too familiar piece can still become an annoyance. If someone is not used to listening for considerable periods of time to music (not just heavy rhythmic or pop songs), do they find some solace in the soothing harmonies and lines of Mozart? Perhaps I need to get out of my small box—to take a break from hearing this kind of music.

D. N. Wheatley, *BipolART*,
DOI 10.1007/978-94-007-4872-9_7, © Springer Science+Business Media Dordrecht 2012

When I take to listening to music seriously again, it is often to Beethoven. He was the finest classical composer, who, through his life, slowly turned to romanticism, with a passion and an emotional tide that few other composers have matched. For me, he was the watershed, the true experimentalist who tried all genres, variations, and even introduced "violations" (discords) so effectively midway through the first movement of the Eroica symphony, that made people sit up and take notice, instead of music up to that time being little more than background (piped) music to calm the nerves of people at grand dinners, etc. But Beethoven made things utterly exciting and incomparable. His genius is always seen through his music—the outward expression of an inward feeling, and one that could not have been other than greatly tormented at times. He may not have been BP, but his mood swings were huge (perhaps within a short time-scale), and his creativity was stupendous. Whether it is music or art, as in putting paint to canvas, one is expressing those innermost feelings which impact massively in such cases on others.

But doodling on musical themes was not impossible during depression; and it seemed to have some therapeutic effect. Some of the following doodles and pictures were done for a particular reason, partly because over the second half of the period being covered (12–13 years), I fell in love with my new partner at a music course in the South of England. She is a professional violinist, and we have been together since 2006.

The set of seven doodles that follow were all drawn in pencil on A4 sheets. Names were given to them almost immediately after they were finished, and the dates on most of them cover the whole period dealt with in this book.

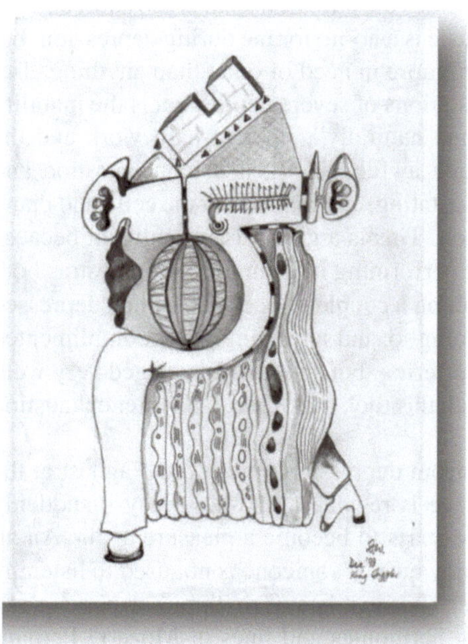

King Juggler (playing castanets; 1999)

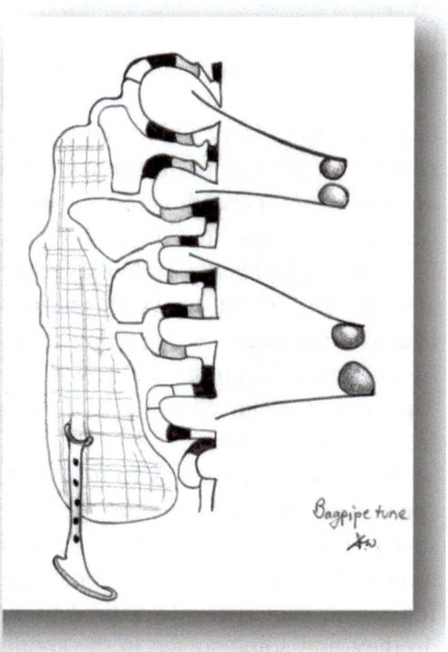

Bagpipe tune (2004)

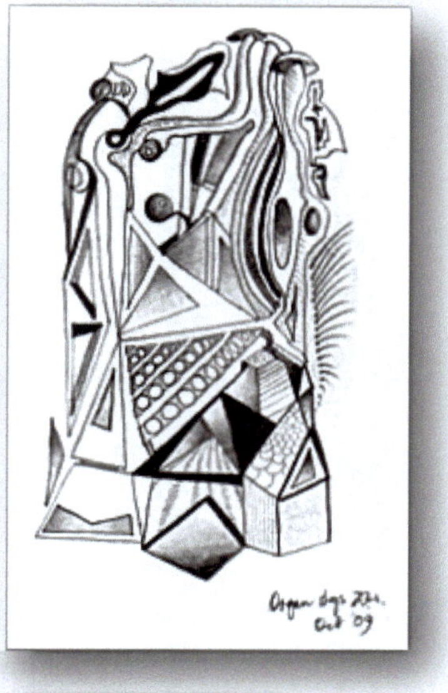

Organ stops (2009)

Many doodles have been produced, however, with some odd motifs, while others are purely about instruments and notes. The majority are pure fantasy, and I have no idea what was in my mind, for example, when a harp-like structure developed balloons on it. The next is like a Scottish leader of a pipe band—the Scottish theme is not that surprising, since I have had a home in Scotland for over 40 years.

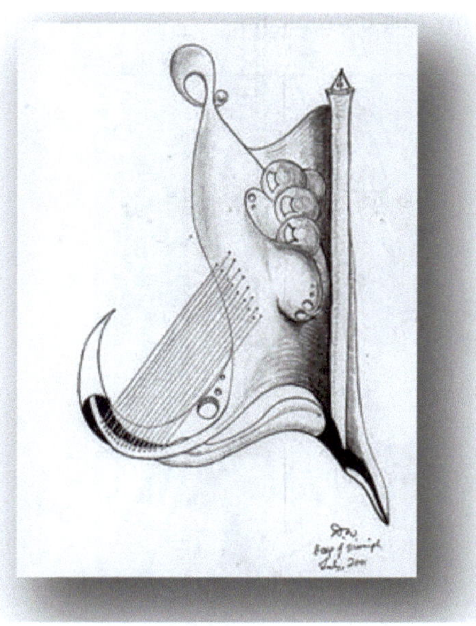

Harp of triumph (2001)

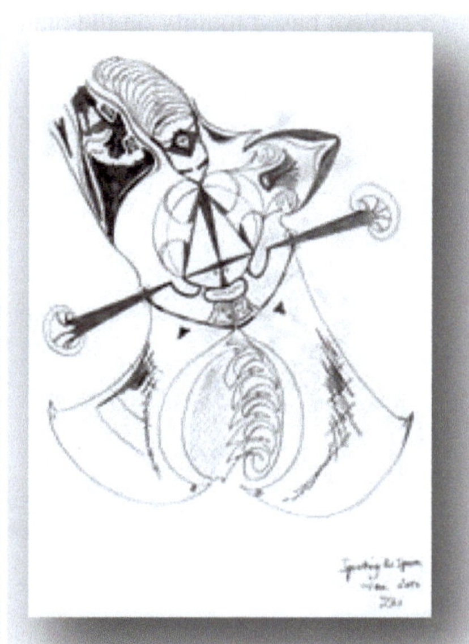

Sporting the sporan – drum major (2000)

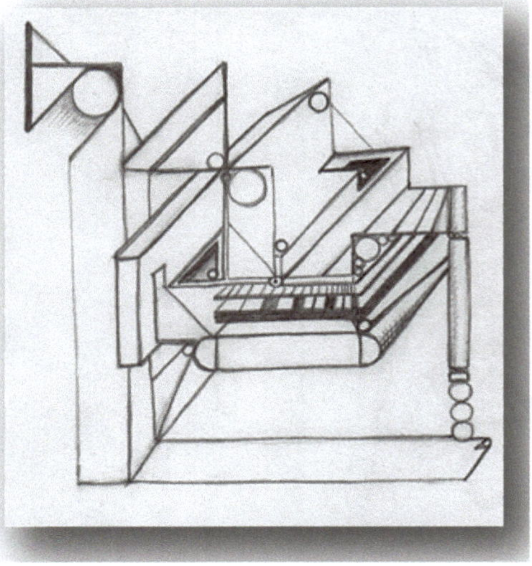

Organ console (2004)

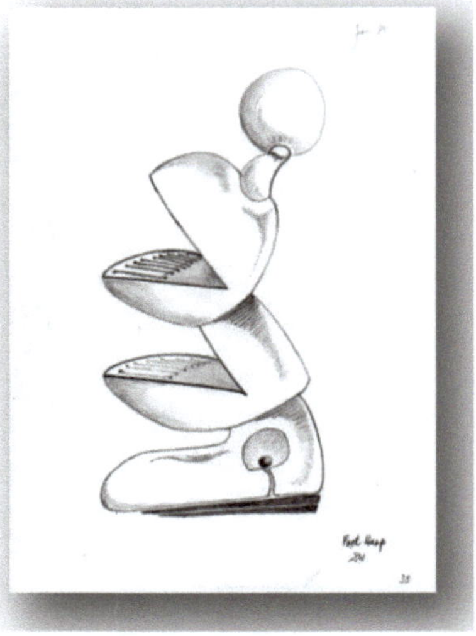

Foot harp (2001)

> Music expresses feeling and thought, without language;
> It was below and before speech, and it is above and beyond all words.
>
> (Roger Ingersoll)

In finding a new partner, not unexpected through my musical connections, I wanted to paint a picture for her that she would like. The following conglomeration of musical paraphernalia came together. While the next painting was done in watercolour, the second picture over the page is a pencil drawing which was seen as more appropriate for a subject based mainly on the piano, my first instrument.

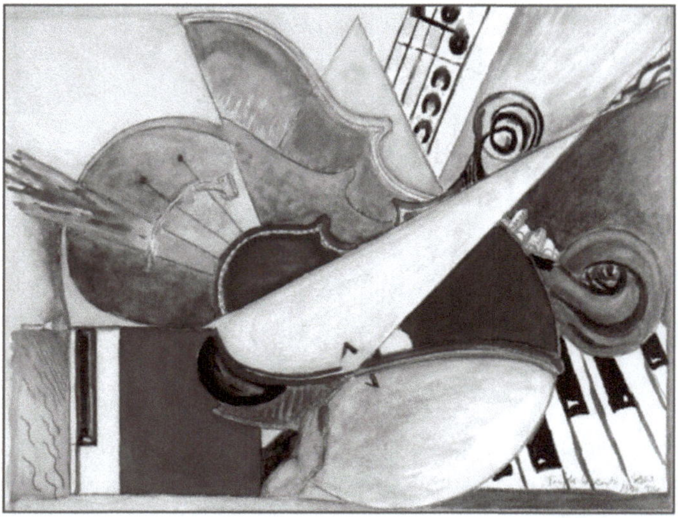

Triple Concerto [1]
Watercolour
November 2004
30 x 21

I especially like this second "triple concerto", and we use it in promotional brochures of the Heller Quartet, led by Jean.

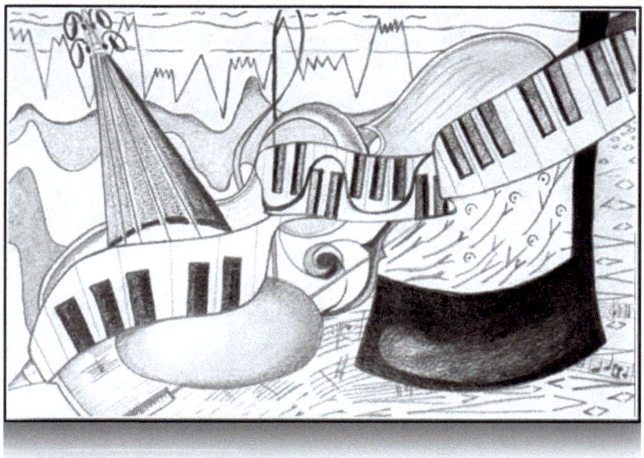

Triple Concerto [2]
Pencil
February 2005
30 x 21

One day during a deep winter depression, while listening to her quartet rehearsing in the house, I decided to make a small sketch of the four instruments. It took no more than about 20 minutes. to complete. I just seemed to fall into place, and I like it probably because of this.

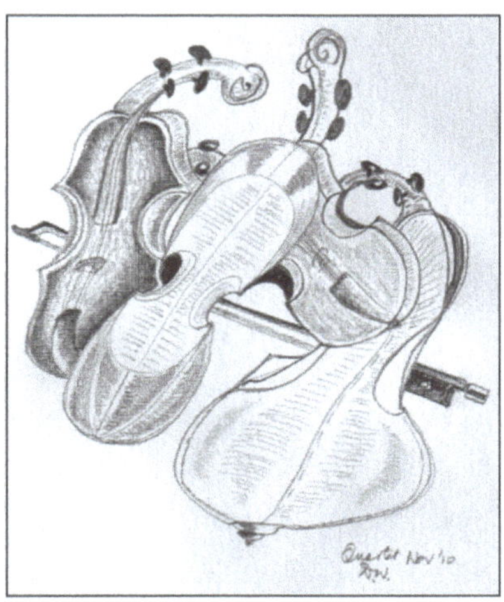

Quartet
Pencil
November 2010
13 x 15

Music alone with sudden charms can bind
The wand'ring sense, and calm the trouble mind
(William Congreve: *Hymn to Harmony*)

Chapter 8
Abstract Art—A Mind Roaming Free

Limitations live only in our minds.
But if we use our imagination, our possibilities become limitless.
(Jamie Paolinetti)

After a particular doodle had been started during a depression in 2002, a new departure crept in which led to some abstract paintings as "themes" over the following years, which I seemed to keep coming back to when a bad depression was definitely lifting and a doodle showed some promise of being a major picture. The four paintings that follow the doodle below show a definite division in the picture between the lighter and darker areas—a reflection of the extremes of BP, a kind of yin-yang (?).

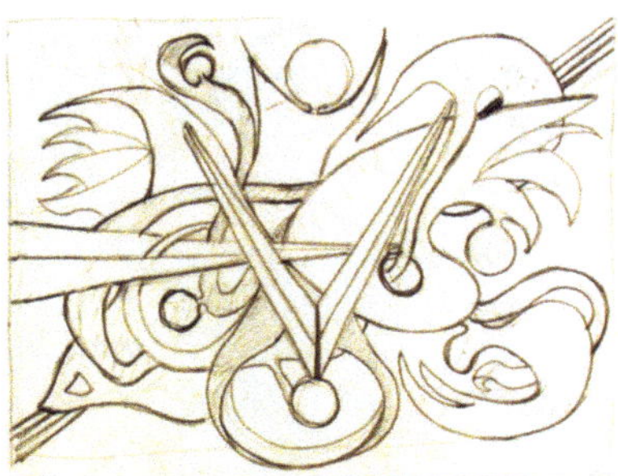

The "division" in this doodle is produced by a sword-like image that extends across the canvas, dividing the blue-sky side from the darkness above (the obverse of how we usually place them), as seen in the picture below. The second picture on the next page, however, has its bright side up.

D. N. Wheatley, *BipolART*,
DOI 10.1007/978-94-007-4872-9_8,

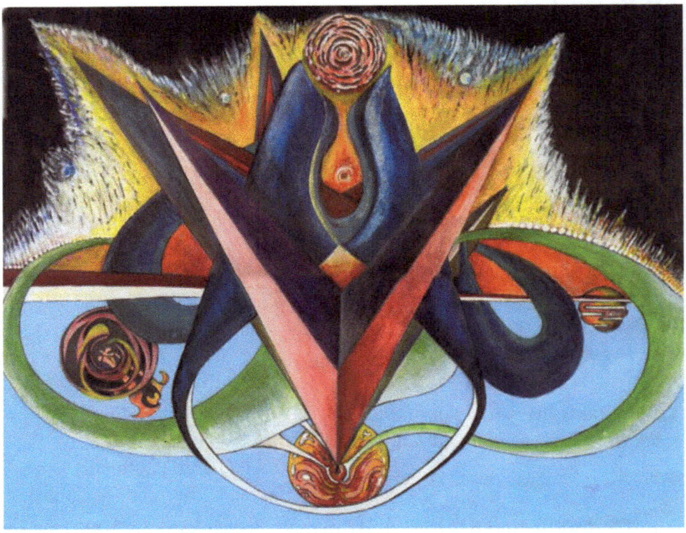

Birth of the spheres
Acrylics
January 2004
40 x 30

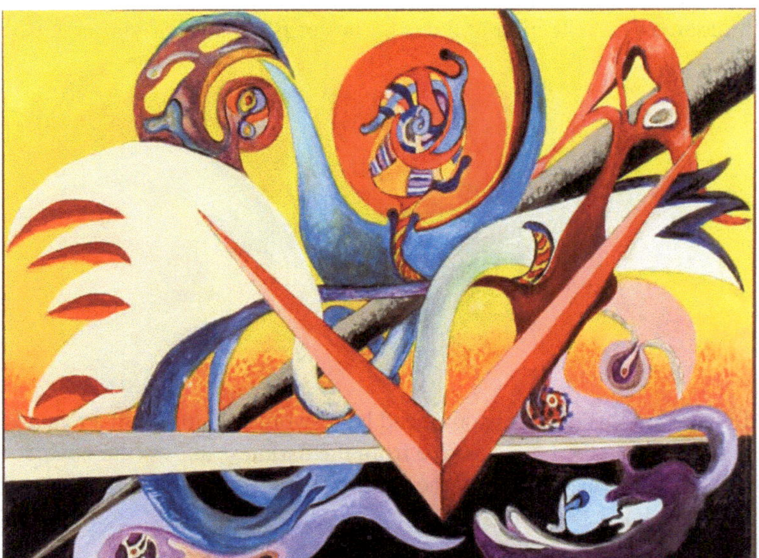

Emergent life
Acrylics
March 2005
30 x 20

The two previous pictures are so similar to one another with that definite theme in mind. That feature can also be seen in the next two images, the dark side now being on top again. This genre of acrylic art continued for a time, but none like it has been done in the last 4–5 years.

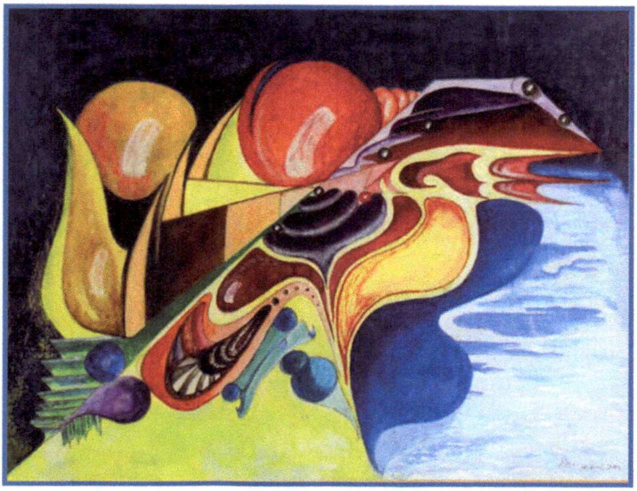

Sea of the Spheres
Acrylics
January 2006
22 x 19

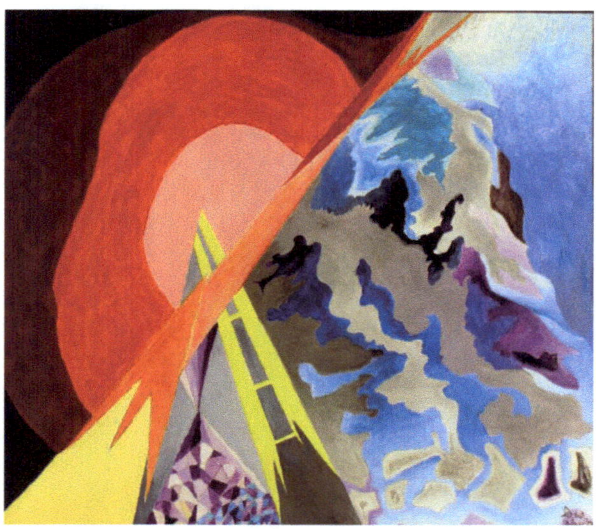

Ascending from the depths
Acrylics
January 2006
22 x 20

Spheres, one of Plato's perfect forms, abound in much of my artwork, but there seems to be a constant questioning of where they come from and how they form. Here's another example with a quadrant-style surround, changing colours in each corner.

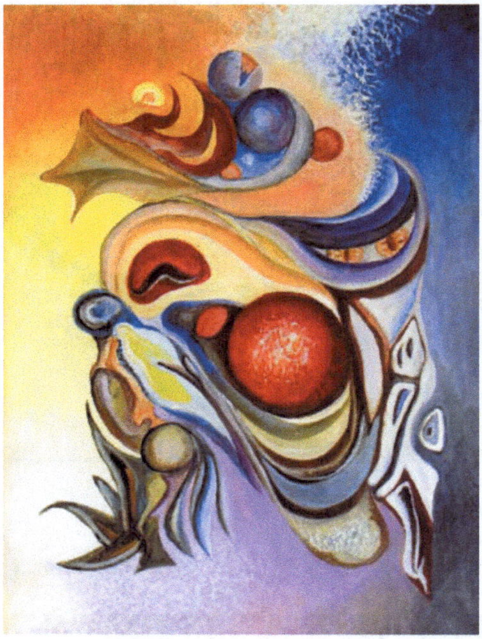

Red centre
Acrylics
March 2008
24 x 40

Spheres stand out in the next image, which is the biggest picture I have ever done.

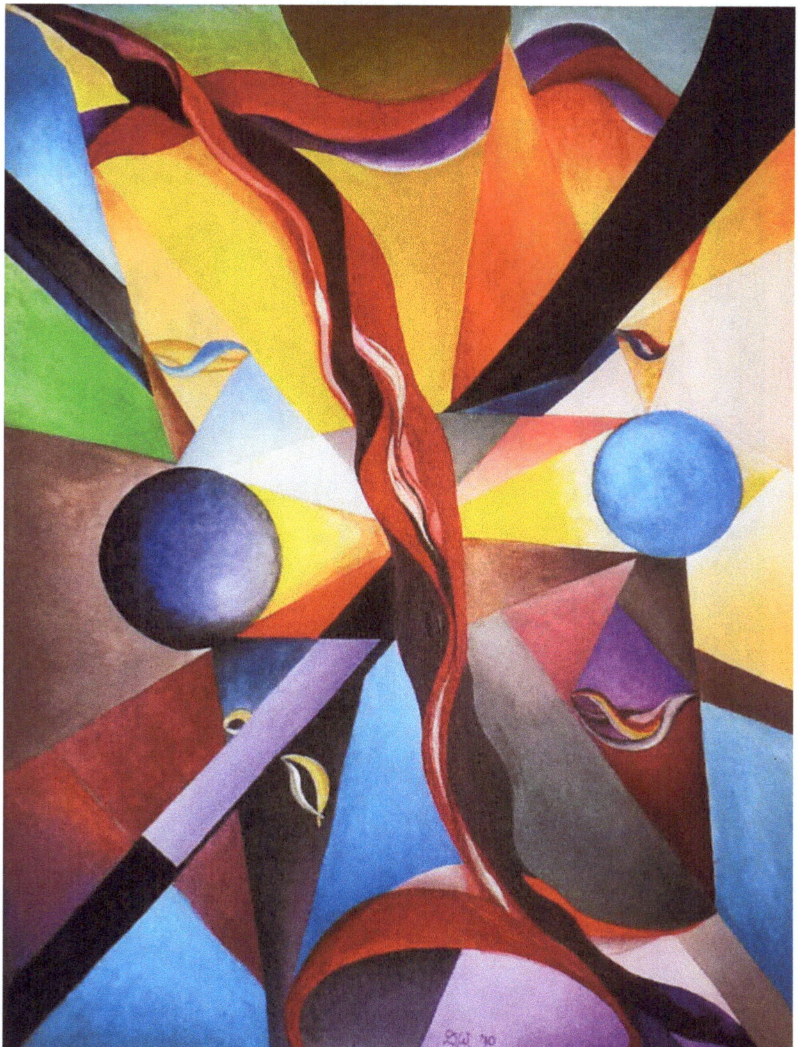

Two spheres
Acrylics
December 2007
55 x 75

The images that follow revolve more around some kind of symmetry. The medium continues to be vibrant acrylics, the next in deep-blue. Many drawings and paintings have lots of compartments in them, often forming spirals, in this case like looking down a spiral staircase.

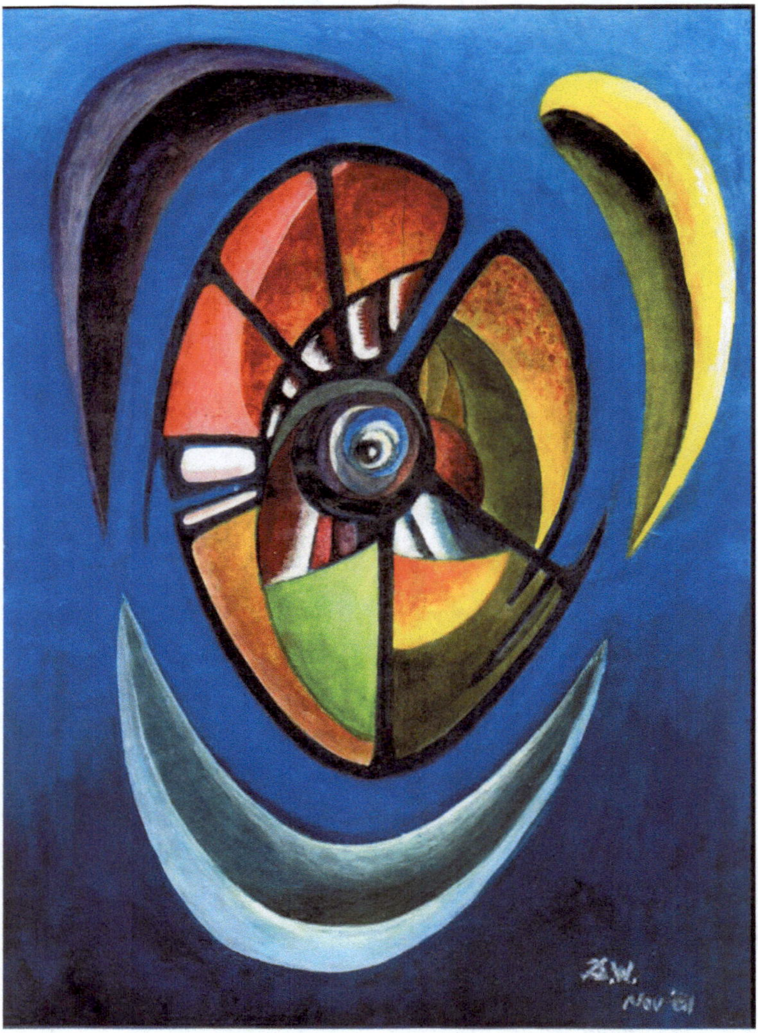

Blue staircase
Acrylics
November 2001
17 x 30

Several pictures remain favourites; there has to be something special about them that tells you (and me, perhaps) a little about the creative mind behind them. The next two are among the best I have produced.

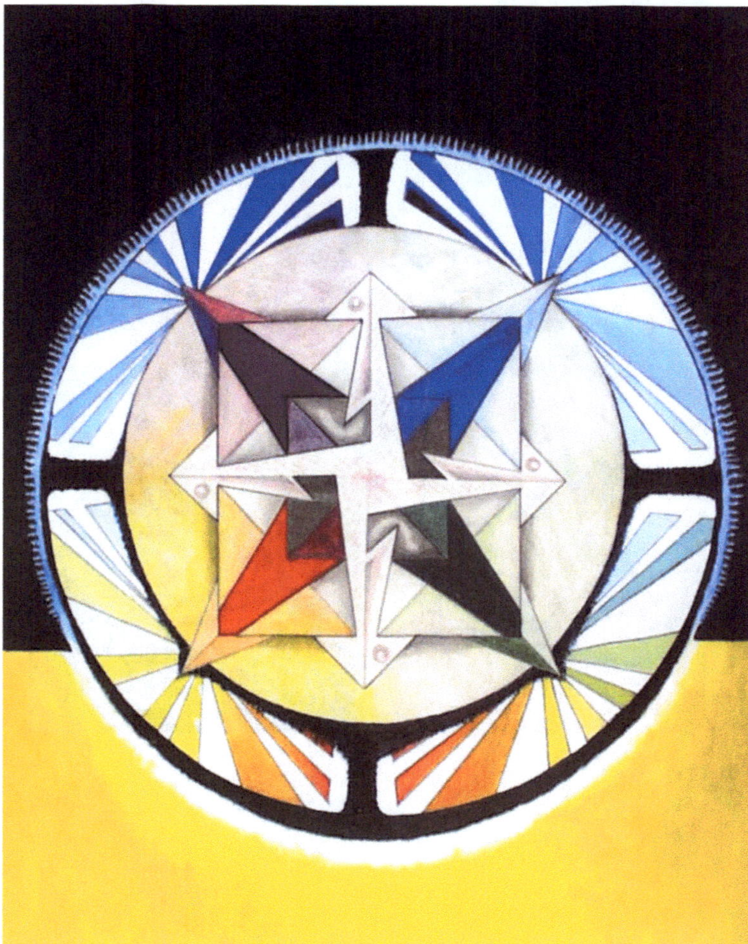

The four winds of colour
Acrylics
March 2001
48 x 54

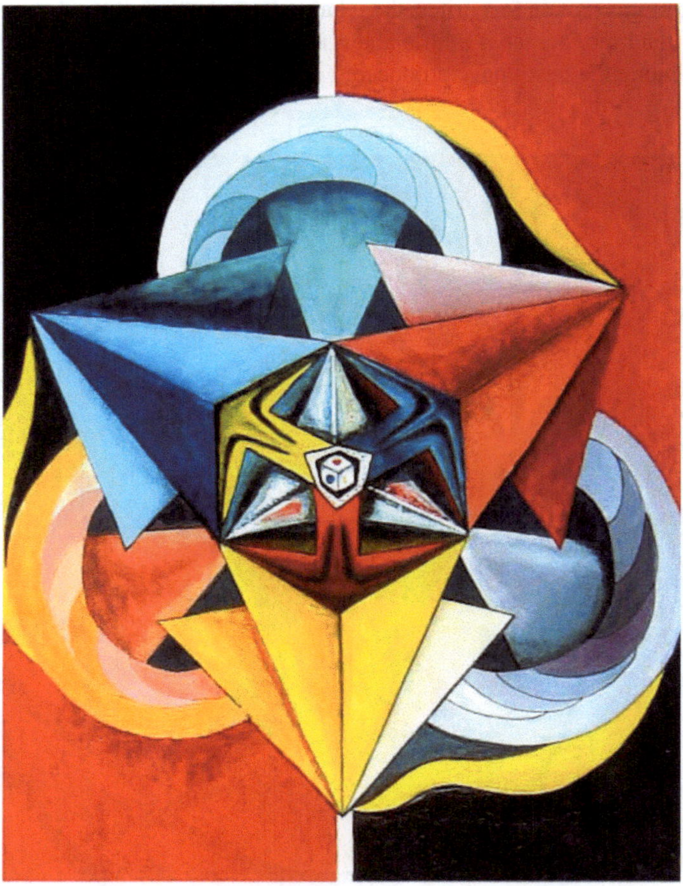

Triome 1
Acrylics
February 2002
24 x 40

Later in the same year after Triome1 had been painted, I produced one ink, one pencil and two coloured images of a similar design. There was undoubtedly an obsession with this intricate mingling of triangles, spheres and cones. Geometry is definitely the force behind this work, as will become evident in a later chapter.

I have not sought to learn (or be taught) new techniques, but sometimes I have been lucky to come across someone to show me other ways of painting and drawing. The technique I used in the next picture was to cover a canvas with water, wipe it gently with a tissue, and drop paint on it from 8 to 10 inches above.The paint can be moved around by tilting the canvas, blowing on it through a straw, or simply pushing it around physically. This painting took less than half an hour, was selected for entry

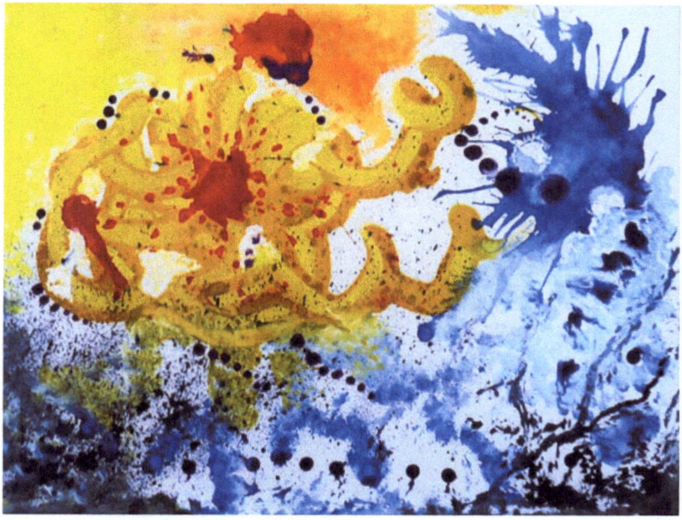

"61"
Water paints
June 2011
40 x 30

into a catalogue for the regional "open studios" week, and was sold to someone who saw it there before seeing the canvas itself, which was quite astonishing. She was taken by the vibrant use of primary colours (which we will have more to consider in the chapter on Geometry). It is called "61" because of the number of blue spots on it, the only part of the whole picture that was deliberately carried out, each dot being placed where I wanted it, in contrast to the randomness or spontaneousness of the rest of it.

Some of my pictures clearly have been influenced by hours spent poring over art books or going around galleries. Fortunately I have travelled widely and seen many of the world's finest museums and art galleries, allowing me to become familiar with many of the greatest works of art ever created. The question always seemed to be the same wherever I have been—what made the artist produce that image, especially when it is an abstract piece? I ask myself, what makes me draw what I draw, but there seldom seems to be any obvious reason.

I have a fondness for the works of Ferdinand Léger, but I did not consciously set out to paint something in his ilk. The hammer-like "pendulum" in this picture smacks of an industrial scene, and portrays something quite different in being much more robust than in many other pictures.

> Lovers and madmen have such seething brains.
> Such shaping fantasies, that apprehend
> More than cool reason ever comprehends.
> (Theseus in *A Midsummer Night's Dream*, William Shakespeare)

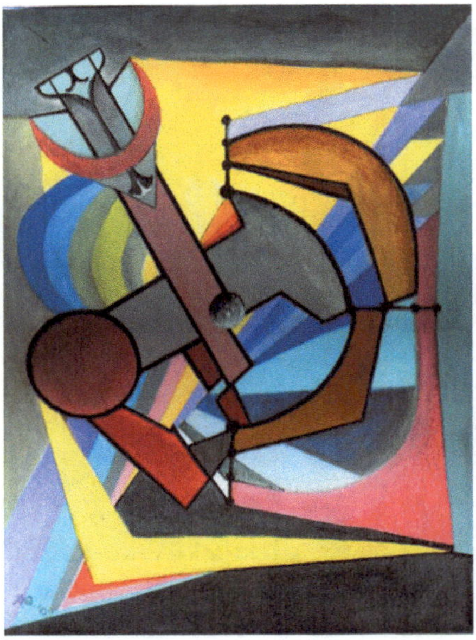

Léger-like
Acrylics
February 2009
30 x 40

Another picture that started with a set of parallelograms in bright colours suggested subsequently to me a beach front setting, an idea that was consolidated by putting the sea in the foreground—I had a Florida (Miami) scene in mind. But there is some real darkness in this otherwise rather gaudy abstraction as can be seen from the purple-black area in the very centre.

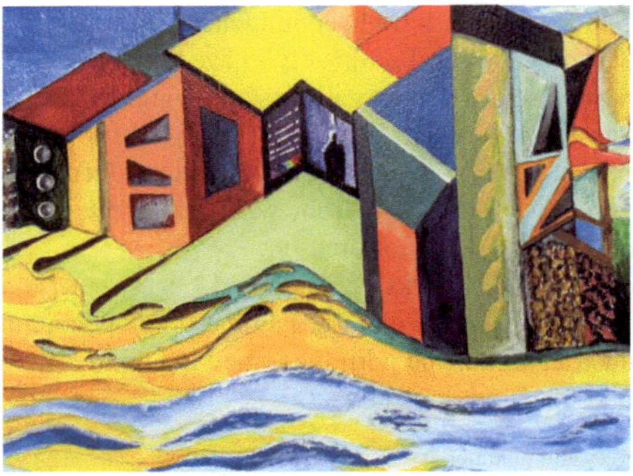

Miami beach scene
Acrylics
March 2007
35 x 24

But another abstract drawing done about the same time contained features that look like a desert with a camel and a cavern in it, but none of this was intentional—it just turned out that way.

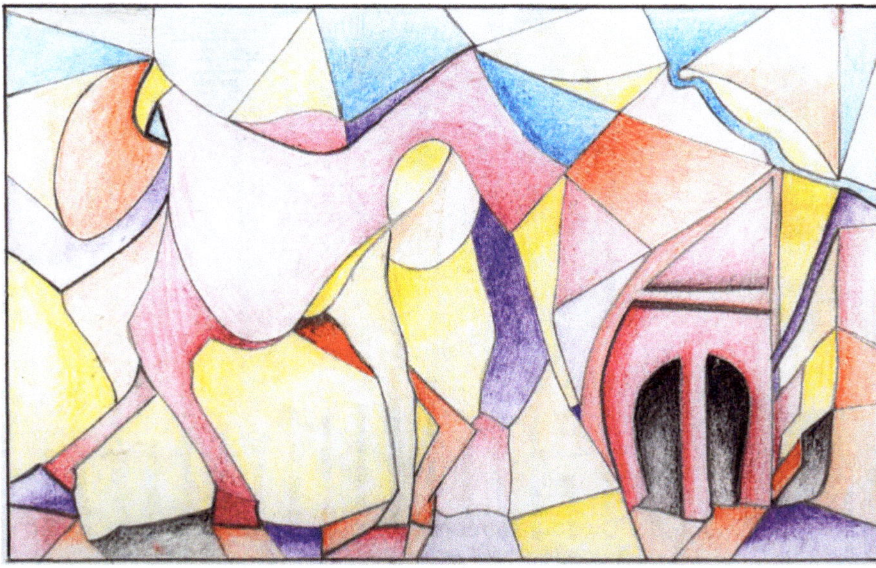

Cave in the desert
Pencil and crayon
February 2007
22 x 14

The next images likewise came out of the blue, but the four elements must have been contrived as a part of my feeling about them in this world. The mural that comes next is a design that I would like to do on a grand scale—a huge wall in a shopping mall or somewhere.

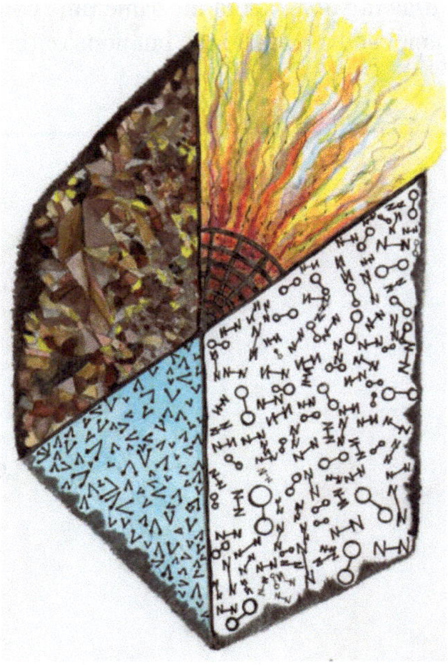

The four elements
Ink and water colour
March 2005
22 x 36

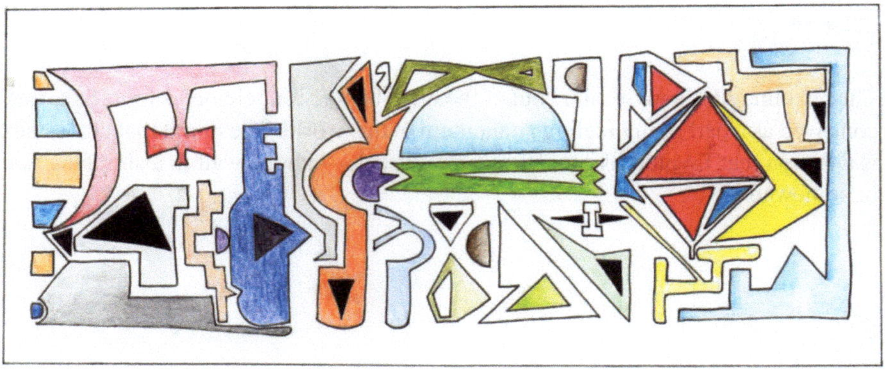

Design for a mural
Pencil and crayon
December 2006
32 x 14

The final picture draws on another famous artist, but of a much different nature. It has the feel of a Rothko picture, an artist who fell into deeper and deeper depression, painting squares with just two colours which became ever darker. This one starts at the top with red life-like bits of tissues and bones, getting paler and squarer as we go downwards, but ending up in purple and finally an almost black rectangle. This picture epitomises depression for me, and it has had a similar feeling on others who have seen it.

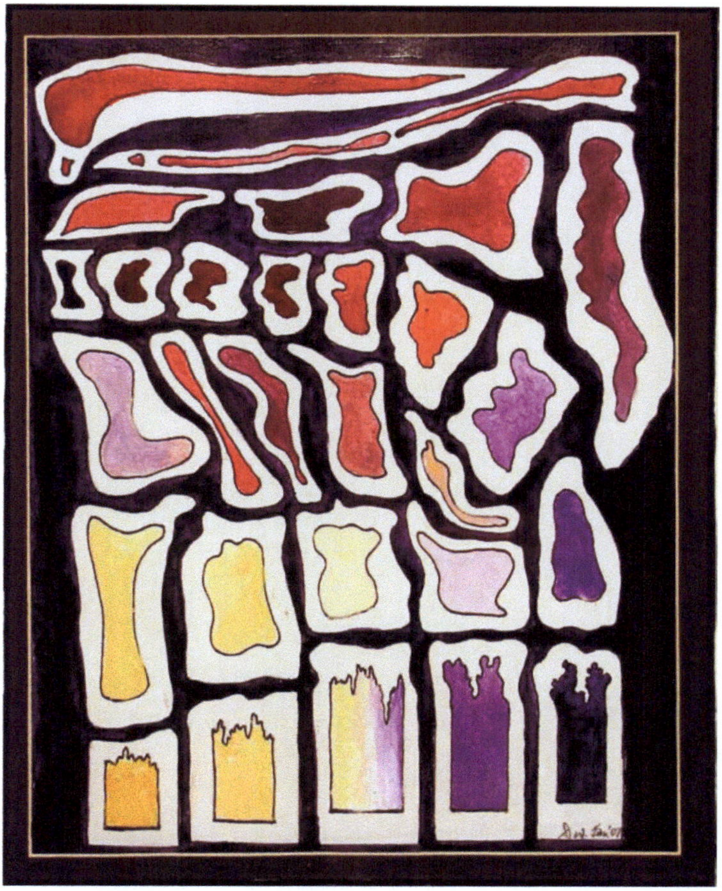

Falling into depression
Acrylics and water colour
January 2007
22 x 35

It's strange how many people suffer from it (fear). I don't mean fear of closed spaces or heights, but fear of death and, what's worst, fear of life.

(Erich Fromm)

Chapter 9
Humour—A Means of Relief

To dry one's eyes and laugh at a fall,
And, baffled, get up and begin again.
(Robert Browning: *Life in a love*)

Another side of BP is mania, during which the sufferer can be very buoyant indeed, laughing and joking as hundreds of ideas flash through the brain, and many associations are made that may be bizarre. There is no question that laughter lightens the mood, lifts life and helps to create real happiness together with others. Laughing is a really phenomenal means of releasing tension; the Dalai Lama suggests we keep smiling, the most gentle and tender way of expressing a state of good humour. It is near impossible to do this in depression, but everyone who gets depressed would be better off if they tried to smile and laugh.

One of my passions in scientific research (truly an obsession) is with a minute submicroscopic organelle of the cell called a "centriole" (Wheatley, 1982). I have spent many hours on long haul flights and other monotonous (even boring) occasions designing innumerable variations on its basic theme. The centriole, despite its size, is truly beautiful in form. It is undoubtedly one of the oldest structures to be found in cells throughout the living world:

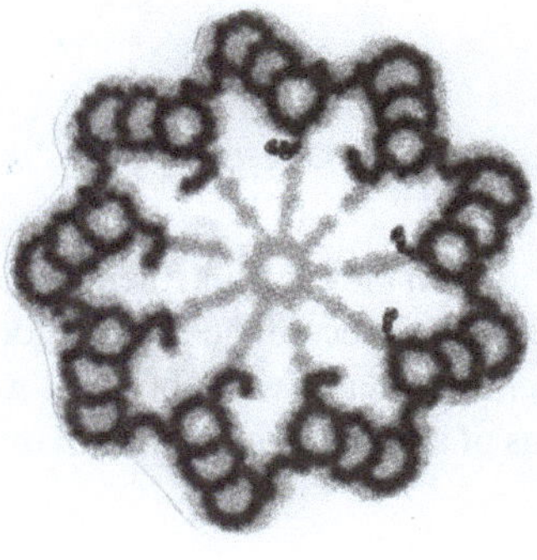

The centriole's 9-fold pattern
(many thousand times magnified)

9-fold symmetry of the Baha'i

D. N. Wheatley, *BipolART,*
DOI 10.1007/978-94-007-4872-9_9, © Springer Science+Business Media Dordrecht 2012

The slant of the triplets in each arm means that it is cannot have perfect symmetry, but it close enough and the whole structure is truly harmonious. Nine is a treasured number in a few cultures, the Japanese being one. A lesser known culture (religion) is that of the Baha'in faith, which adopted the ninefold symmetrical symbol above as its emblem—underlining the beauty of the lotus flower. One of the temples of the Baha'ian faith in Chicago uses this design. The unfolding of its nine petals is a motif that permeates much of the art and craft work of the Orient.

The basic design of the centriole can be manipulated in many artistic ways, but I always gave a lot of thought to each one to try to make them as interesting as possible, with apt titles. It has been a game I have been playing for many more years than I have been covering in this book, so in this sense I now have to admit that have been indulging in a form of doodling for about 20–30 years. This activity has a definite goal and cannot therefore be the classical doodling that comes from spontaneous drawing. The motif of the three circles (tubules) making up each arm can be seen all over the place in life, and then it is a matter of fitting them into the complete pattern. For example, the three sections of an insect body, the ant, can make up the three tubules. By linking nine ants up, I created one of the first variations on the theme. A similar variation can be made with a clone of fat mice, used as a model of obesity in scientific research.

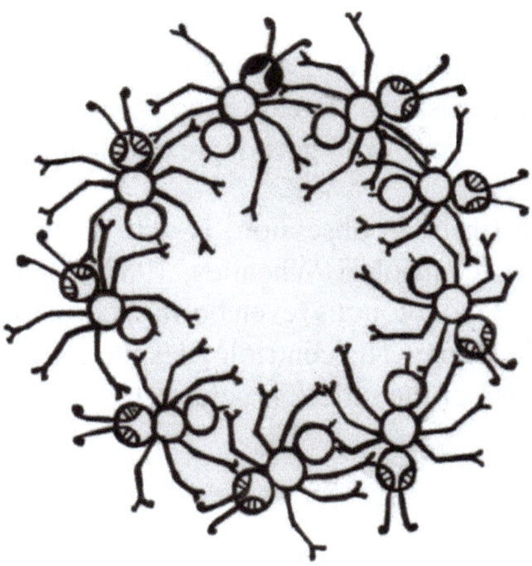

Ants – clone, with dark-eyed mutant

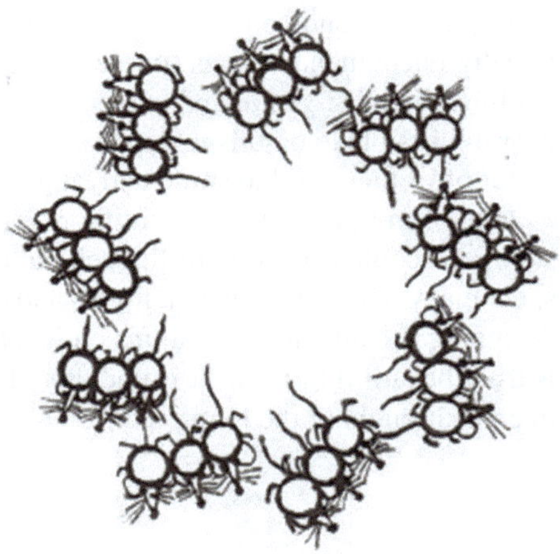

Obese mice

In all I have created about 80 different variations on the centriole theme, and throughout I have striven to produce humorous ones. It has been done in both good and bad times, but more often in the former, and certainly has always brought with it light relief in one way or another—a simple means of amusing oneself! But I do hope they may also bring a smile to your face.

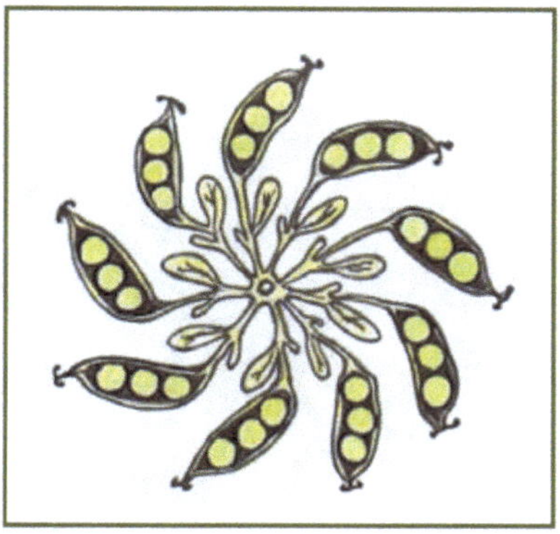

Homage to Mendel, the father of genetics (Peas - *Pisum sativum*)

Setting out the pints of dark beer almost got me into a dispute with Guinness, who thought the next doodle on the centriole was too close to their (then) promotional campaign. But the glasses might not be filled with their stout, and they cannot claim to have monopoly of the word "genius".

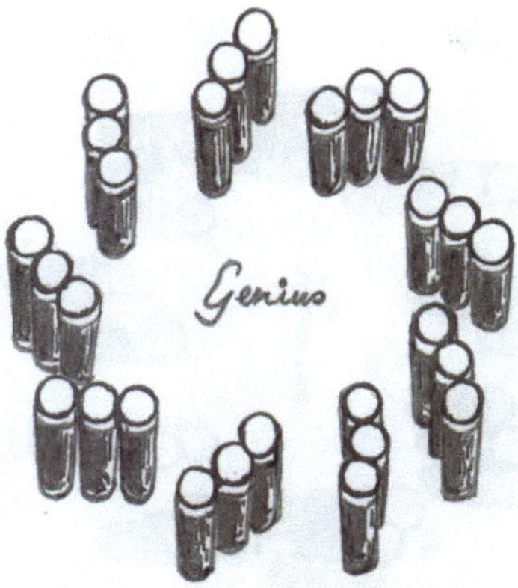

Pints of beer

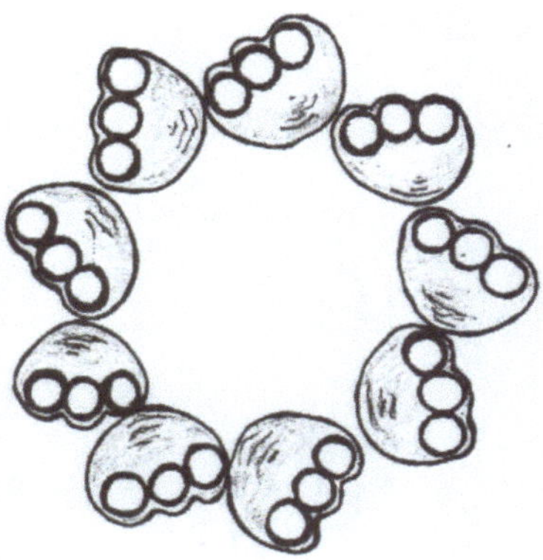

Elephant toes

It just happened one day that I noticed the feet of elephant and found their three toe nails would fit the pattern. In another doodle (not shown), I used big elephant ears with the head in the middle to fit the triplets—it's amazing how many things can fit-or can be made to fit- the pattern, for example, the three wheels at the back of HGVs, or the three lights we all see at traffic lights.

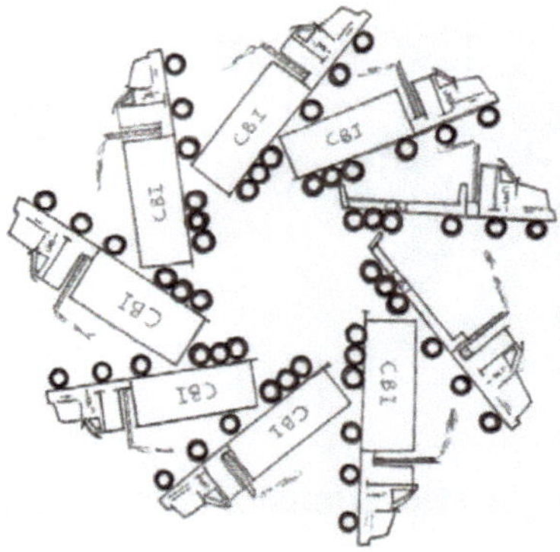

HGV wheels

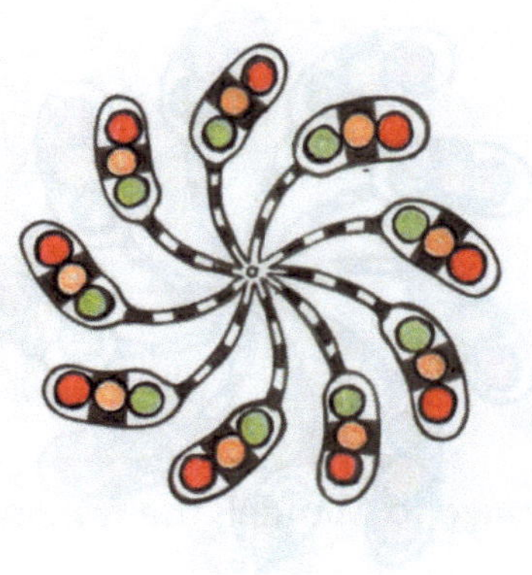

Traffic lights

Some might see the centriole pattern in the gas-burner on the kitchen hob, but with more contriving, it is possible to get Newton's cradles to oblige.

Fruit also lend themselves to the centriole design, cherries and tomatoes.

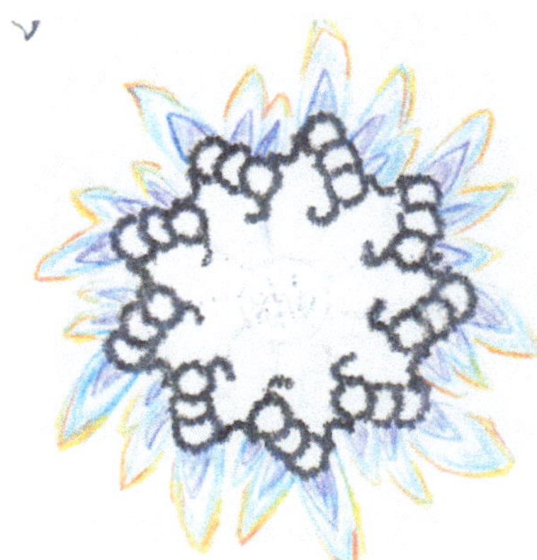

Gas-burner

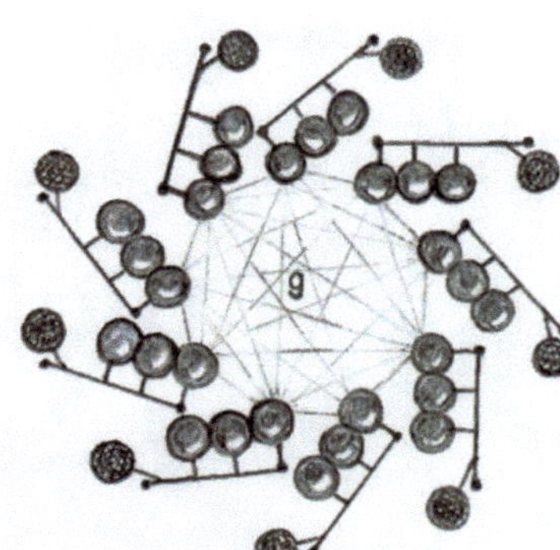

Newton's cradle

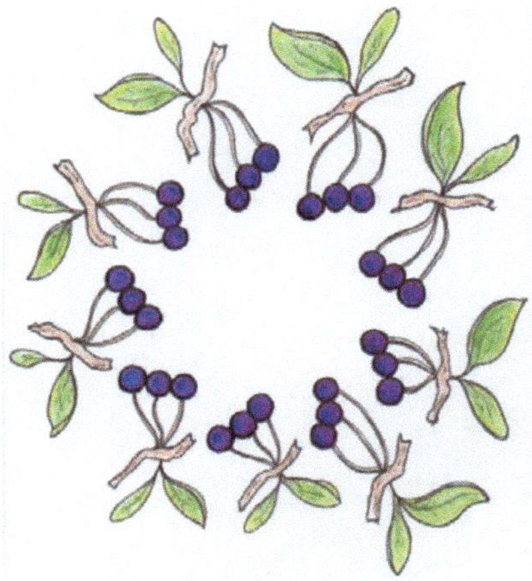

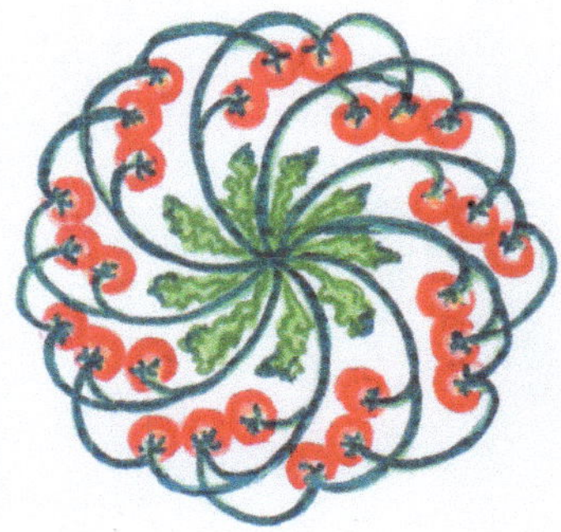

Cherries **Tomatoes on the vine**

And finally, it is possible to depict the centriole in forms of art found in different cultures—this one is done in the aboriginal idiom. I have been working on one based on the tiling patterns of Islamic mosques

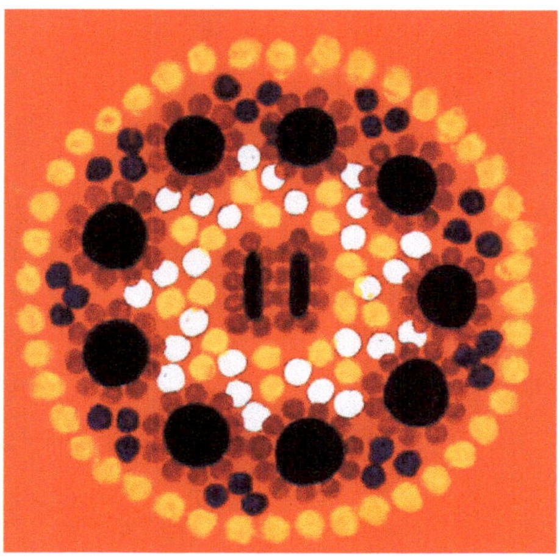

Chapter 10
Goaded by Geometry

Geometry (which is the only science that it hath pleased God hitherto to bestow on mankind).

(Thomas Hobbes: *Leviathan*)

Geometric form has always fascinated me; although it is mathematically based, I cannot by any stretch of the imagination consider myself adept at mathematics. Calculus leaves me cold, but geometry introduces theorems—and to a scientific mind (even from the early inquisitiveness of youth), this calls for proofs, findings ways of establishing the congruence of one thing to another, like the volume of a sphere in relation to its diameter. It creates the basis of all science, the solving of problems by deductive and inductive thinking. So it is no surprise that it has intrigued and fascinated me, although I remain a novice with regard to its application.

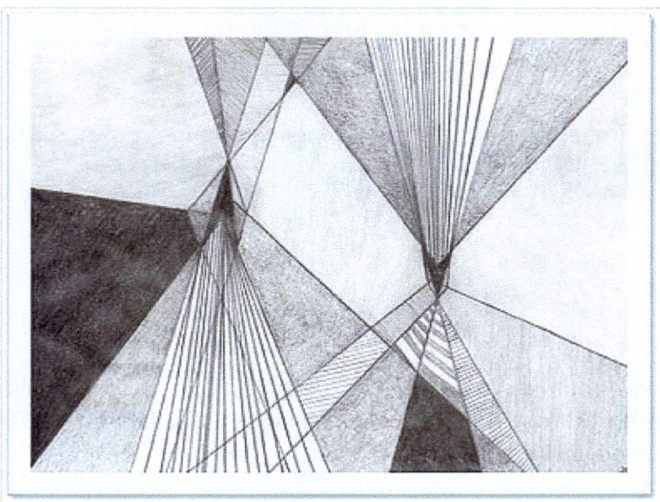

Flypast
Pencil
January 2006
20 x 16

D. N. Wheatley, *BipolART*,
DOI 10.1007/978-94-007-4872-9_10, © Springer Science+Business Media Dordrecht 2012

Most of my doodles are drawn in freehand, but geometry usually demands straight lines and a ruler is more often than not necessary, as you can see from the first picture, which is supposed to depict two high-speed aircraft passing one another.

Shading allows depth to develop from otherwise flat surfaces, and much of Euclid is based on 3-D forms, especially the cone (conic sections). Shading gives lots of different textures, as we see in the next image.

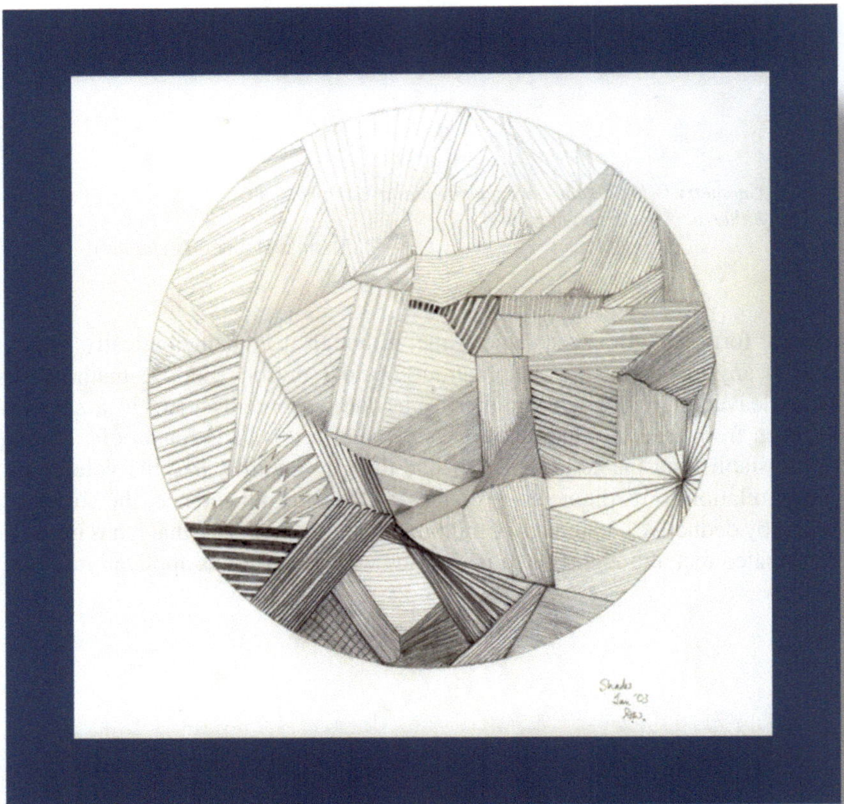

Shades
Pencil
January 2003
30 x 30

It is not surprising then to mix the angular with the conical and spherical, as in the picture that follows. Spheres, cones, triangles and other distinct forms feature frequently in other chapters.

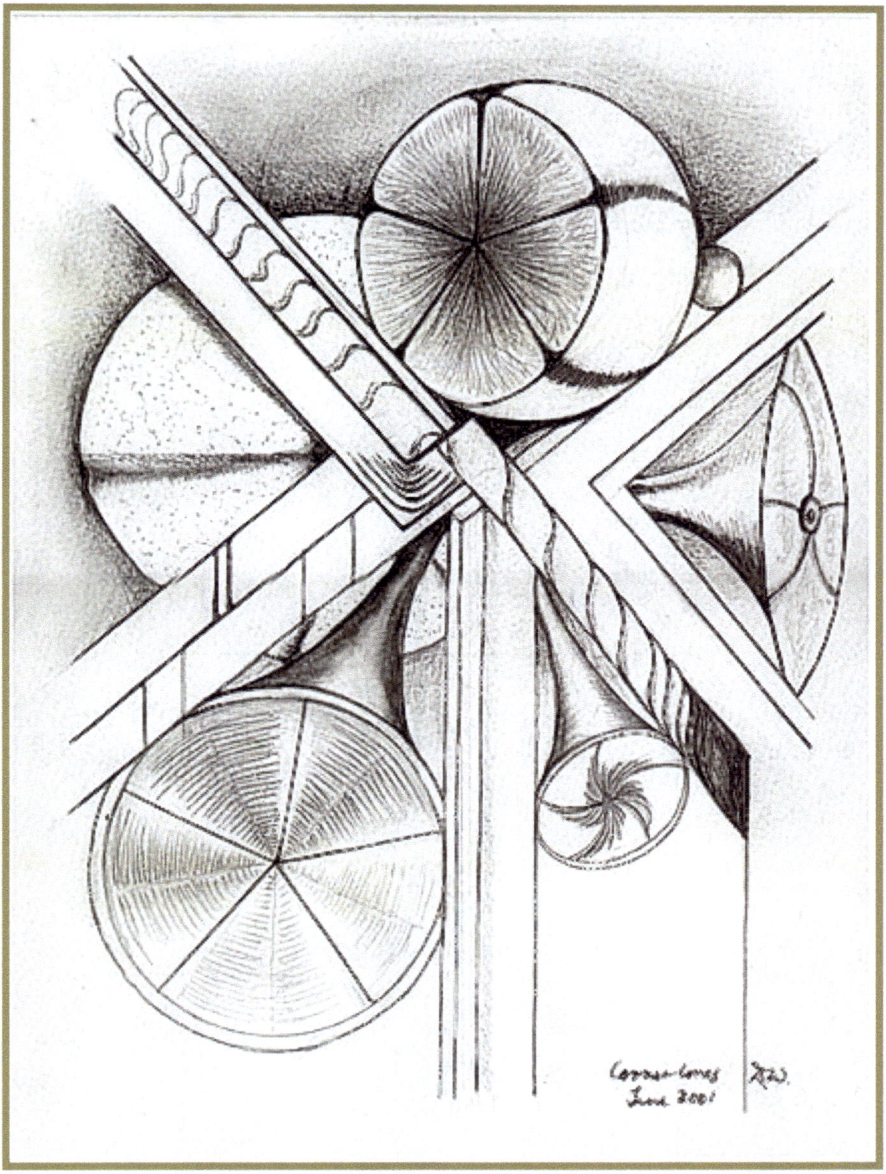

Corner cones
Pencil
June 2001
16 x 26

The stark form of geometry fits uncomfortably within more natural scenes, as in the weird apparition of the structure next seen on what looks like the beach (Compare doodle on page 14). The smaller doodle that follows has a similar juxtaposition. Perhaps bipolarity is expressed in a mixture of the sharp and angular contrasting with the curvaceousness of nature?

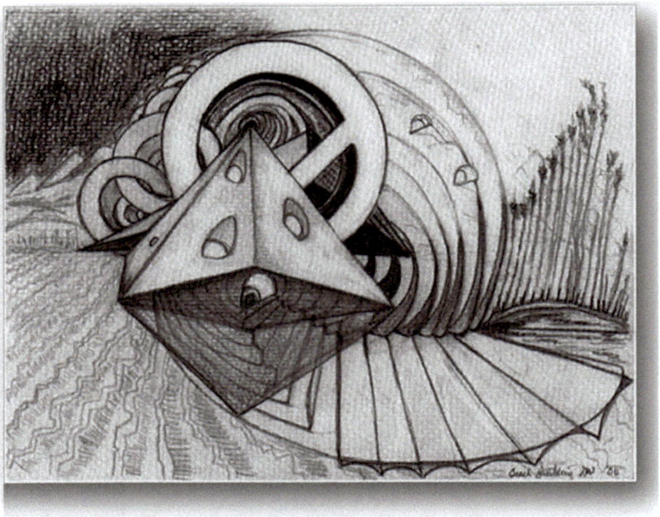

Beach Building
Pencil
January 2004
17 x 12

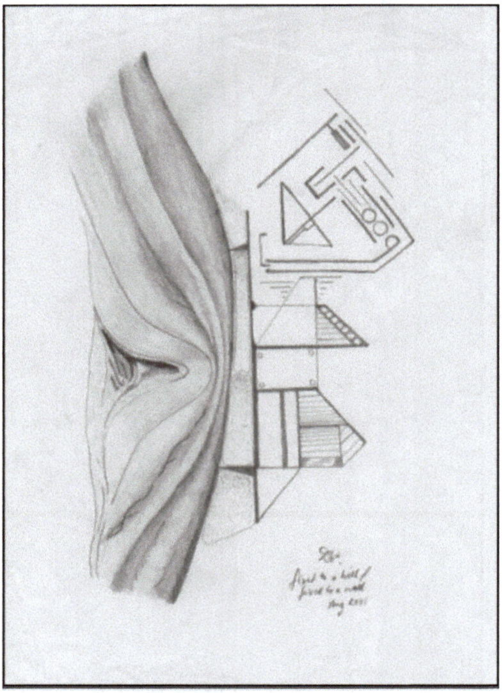

Fixed to a Hill/Fixed to a Wall
Pencil
August, 2001
7 x 10

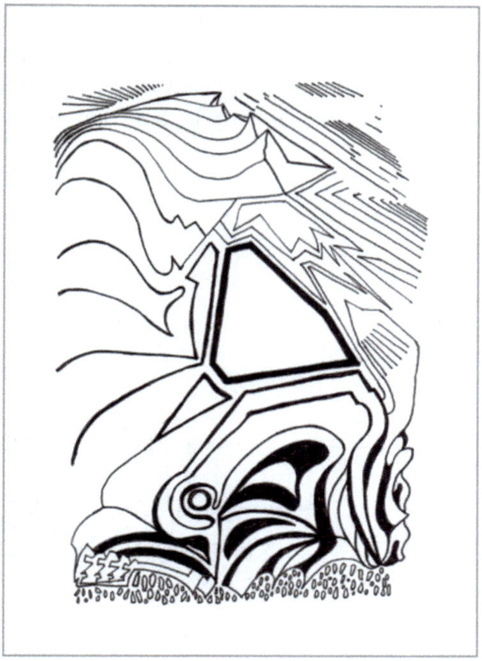

Starkvistas
Indian Ink
December 2009
9 x 14

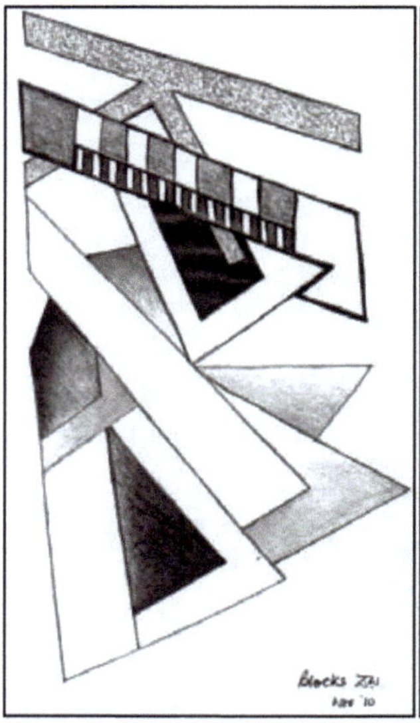

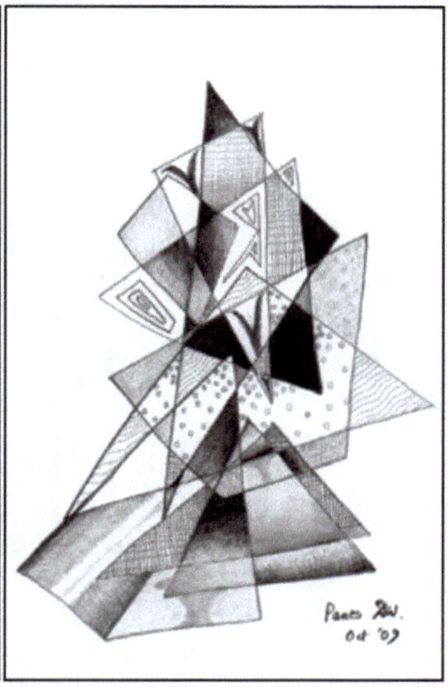

Blocks
Pencil
December 2010
7 x 10

Panes
Pencil
October 2009
8 x 10

The industrial plant is an old doodle that was made as square as possible, the only curves being the faint outline of hills behind. About the same time, a desert scene with a strange engine was drawn. I have no idea what brought these two similar (to me) doodles together. It's the stark geometry in them that makes me include them in this chapter.

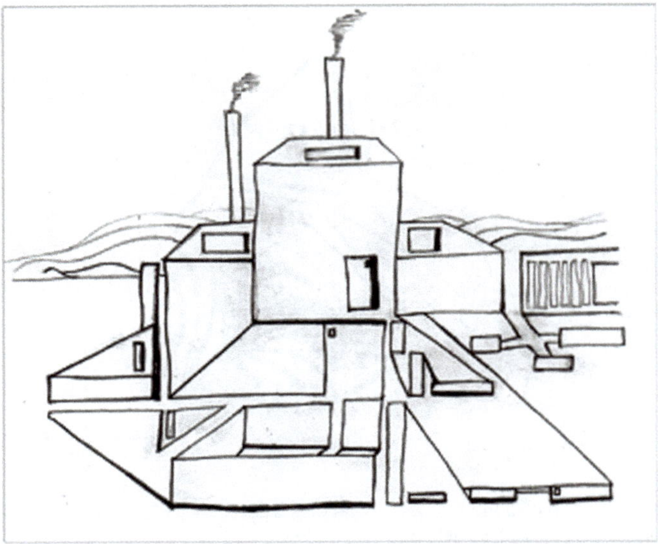

Plant
Pencil
November 2006
13 x 11

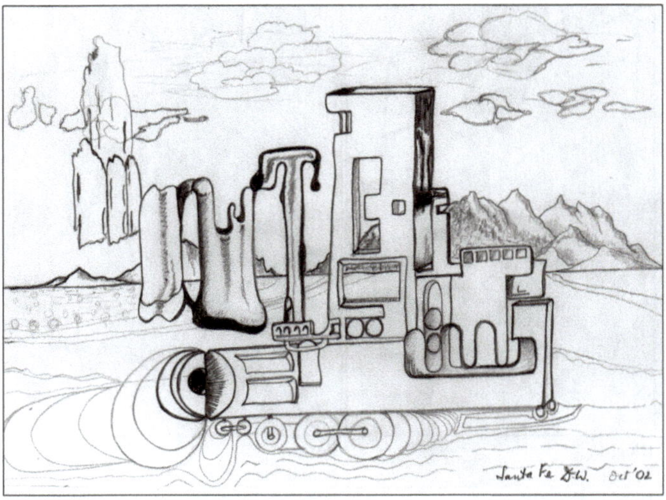

Santa Fe
Pencil
October 2002
20 x 14

An industrial theme seemed to prevail, with a pump having a curving tube through it.

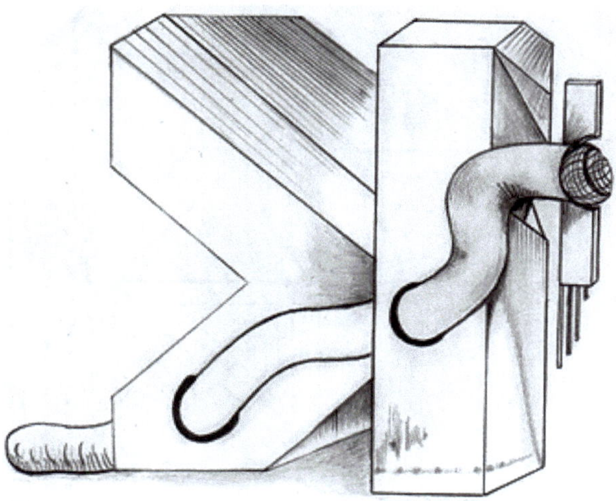

Pump
Pencil
December 2006
12 x 11

But triangles became another theme (obsession?)...

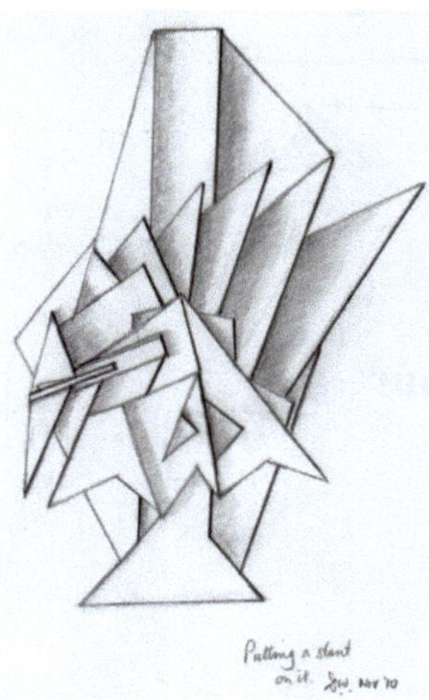

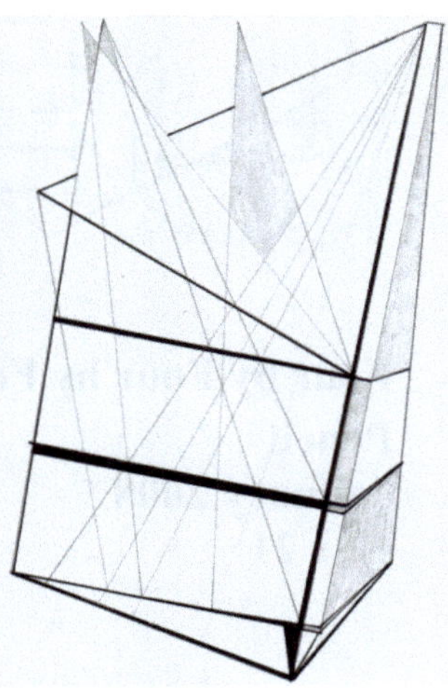

Putting a slant on it
Pencil
November 2010
9 x 15

Suspended form
Pencil
December 2010
11 x 18

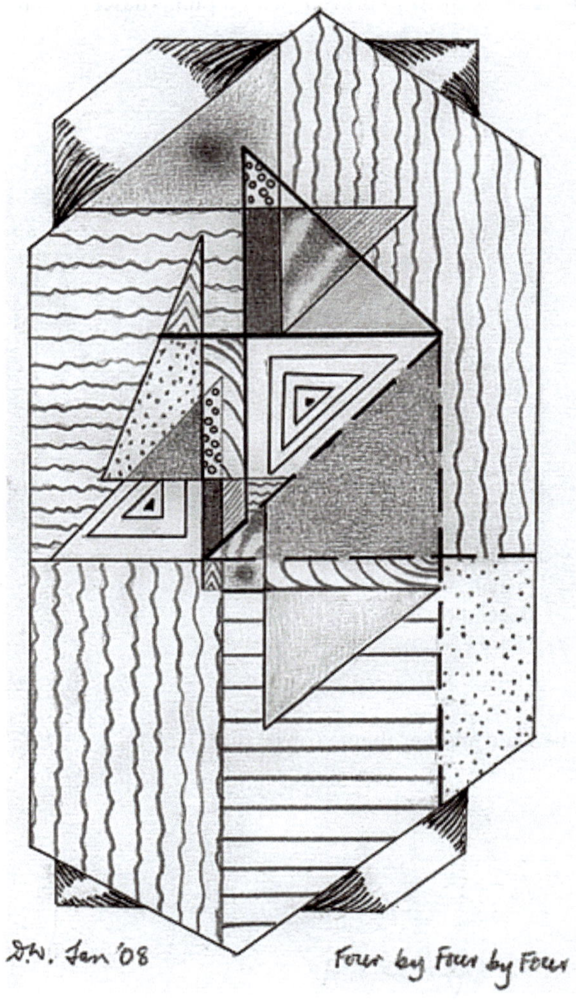

Four by Four by Four
Pencil
January 2008
12 x 21

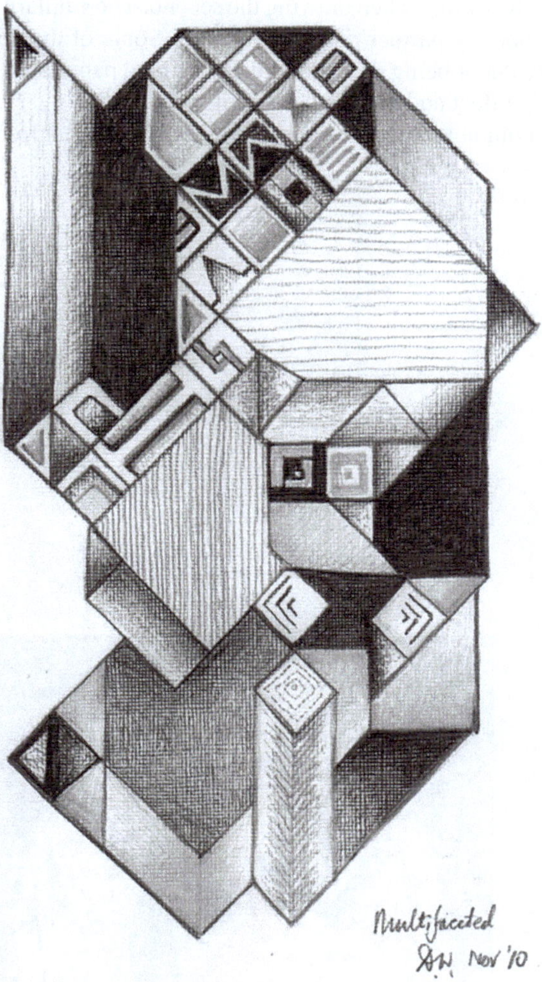

Multifaceted
Pencil
November 2010
11 x 19

The two doodles above were done almost 2 years apart, but I had no conscious recollection of the former when drawing the second. The similarity was only brought home to me when my partner remarked upon it. Some of the textures of the right-hand image are due it being drawn on thick cartridge paper used for watercolour; it gives a pleasing effect and now I often use it.

And oddly I did not seem to be able to get away after that from this design.

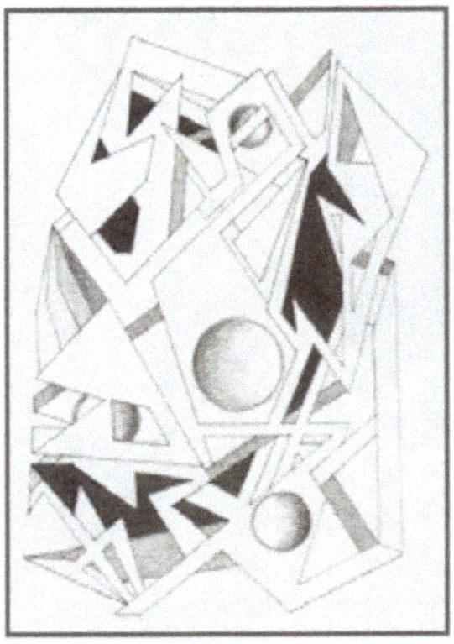

(The original doodle)

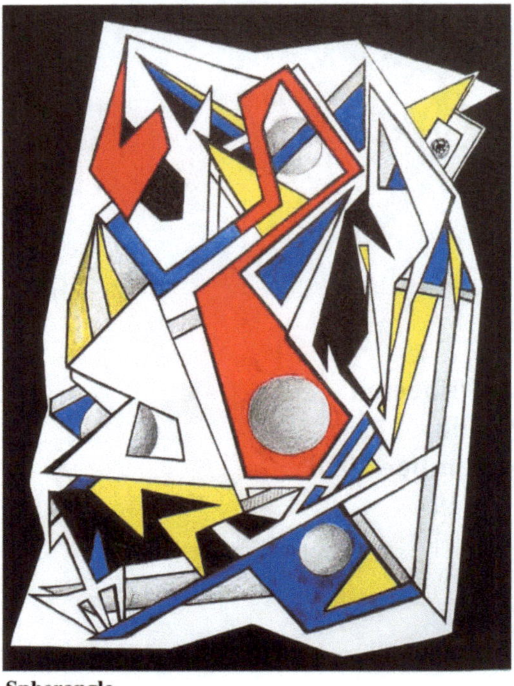

Spherangle
Black ink, pencil and acrylic
January 2011
38 x 48

But this went much further with coils and loops coming among angles, cones and spheres. Projections and grid-like constructions also emerged. . . with this next one done earlier in this series, which had already included a mixture of angularity, with spheres and other shapes in it.

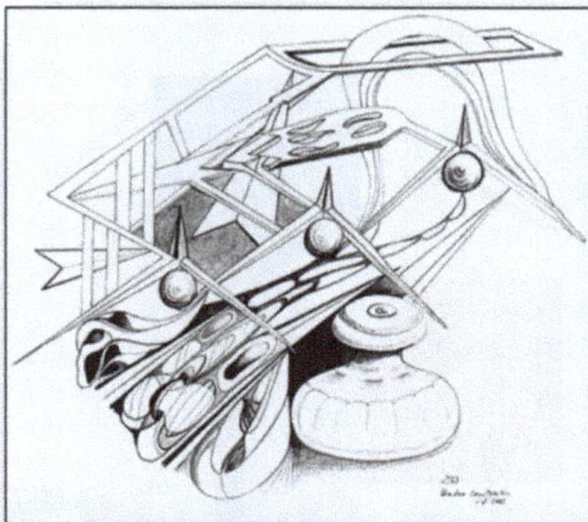

Under Construction
Pencil
September 2003
35 x 26

Even a human form emerged from the angular world of geometry—very much like "Panes" seen on page 95.

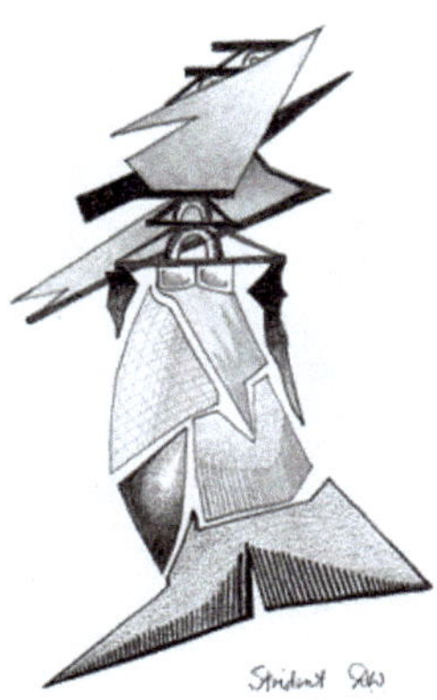

Strident
Pencil
october 2009
8 x 12

While I had only a moderate liking for Mondrian to begin with, I reached the point where I felt that his use of primary colours and straight line geometry could be manipulated to give some more interesting effects than an obsession with the rectilinear grid, naturally with a few spheres added to some of them. The results are the following pictures.

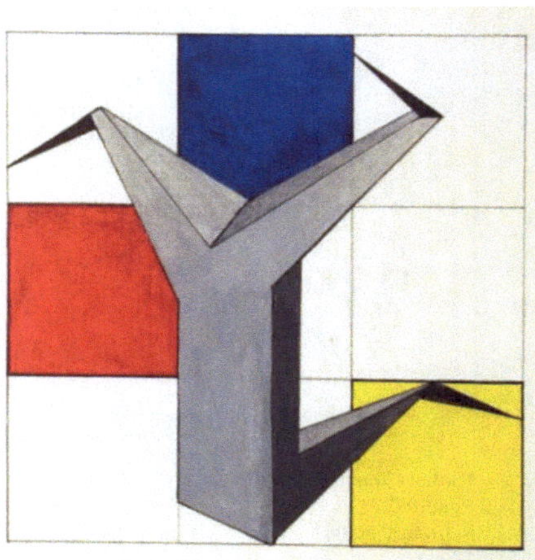

Mondrian Steel
Watercolour, Pencil and Black Ink
December 2006
14 x 14

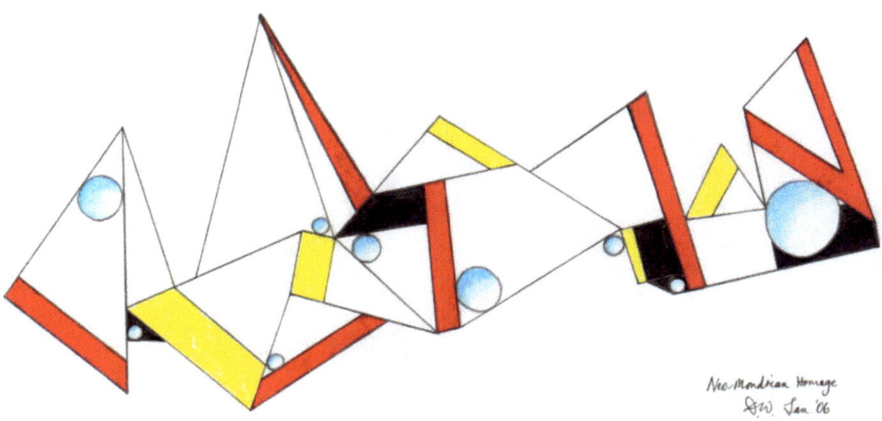

Neo-Mondrian homage
Watercolour and Pencil
January 2006
23 x 12

Playing a further game with Mondrian, I thought I would detach the central square of a typical picture in his style and imagine an invisible ball had been dropped near the middle—to give an Einsteinian curved space-time effect.

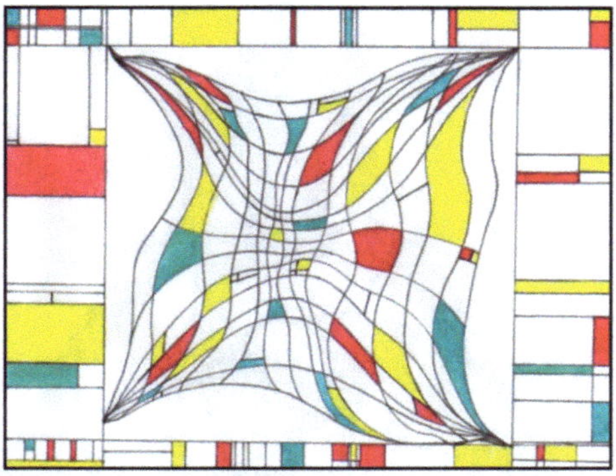

Space-time boogie-woogie
Watercolour and Indian ink
January 2006
14 x 10

To end this part of the gallery, we return to symmetry (or near symmetry), often seen in geometrical forms. This next image is only symmetrical, in some respects, underpinned by a sixfold outline—is this back to the chemistry of the benzene ring of my early scientific training?

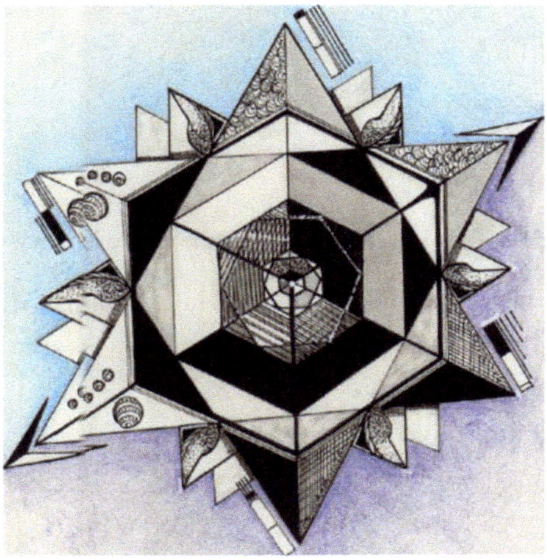

6-Fold "symmetry"
Ink and crayon
December 2005
17 x 17

The drawing below plays with shapes with different numbers of surfaces—1, 2, 3 and 4, and centrally it contains an old design in fivefold symmetry.

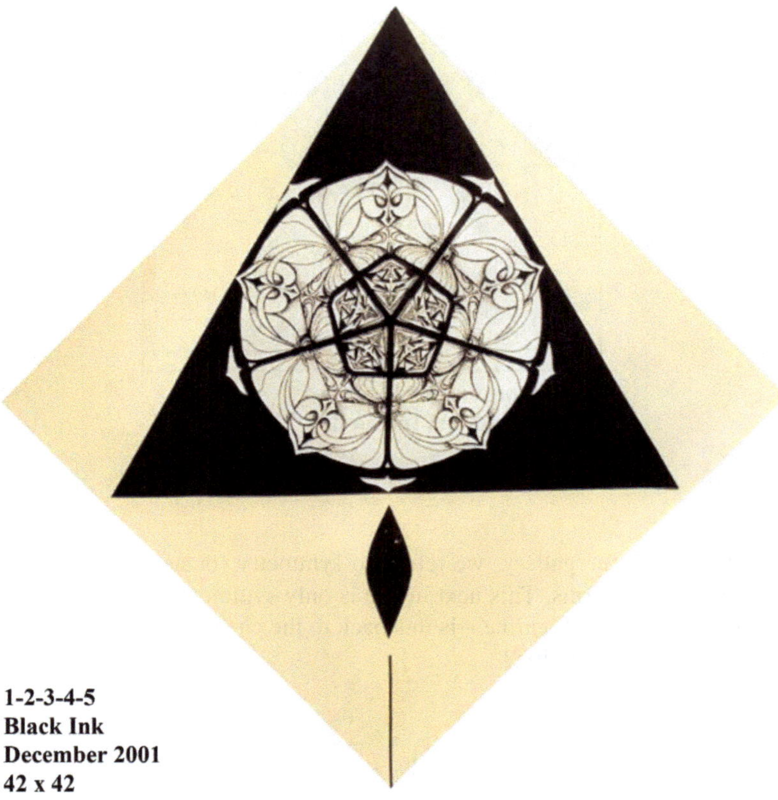

1-2-3-4-5
Black Ink
December 2001
42 x 42

The nature of God is a circle of which the centre is everywhere
And the circumference is nowhere.

(Attributed to Empedocles)

Chapter 11
Epilogue: Art, Creativity and Bipolar Disorder

I sometimes wonder how all those who do not write, compose, or paint manage to escape the madness, the melancholia, the panic fear which is inherent in the human situation

(Graham Green)

The Person(ality) Behind the Art

This book is a personal account and commentary through art, and to a lesser extent by way of the written word, on living with Bipolar Affective Disorder. We all see things subjectively and uniquely, and my account of it will be different from accounts from many other people. Yet humanity is bound together by feelings, emotions and behaviour, all of which are needed for a gregarious species to thrive. I do not wish to bare my soul (mind) as I continue to cherish my privacy; it is clear to many of my friends and acquaintances that I do not often wear my heart on my sleeve. However, there are many aspects of living with BP that I would wish to share with other people, provided they are prepared to listen. Starting with an art show might be a suitable opening—an ice-breaker that then gets the interested party to enter into some serious dialogue about BP. [I have had three one-man shows to date at local venues.] This approach might reduce the tension between those of us afflicted and those around us who at times wonder what on earth is going on, as epitomised in Caroline Carr's book *Living with the Black Dog* (Carr, 2007). The stigma of mental disturbances are becoming much better tolerated by the rest of society as we learn more about mental disorders and their causes; but that stigmatization is still there when affliction is severe. Any action that can reduce it is welcome; after all, who among us can claim to be completely normal?

BP has impacted on my life as a whole, and notably in my dealings in science, medicine and art, and these aspects can be shared with you through different parts of this epilogue. I trust that the pictures will have given you a little insight into the personality behind them—that was the prime intention in writing this book. However, the nature of that personality needs to be exposed more fully now if what I have done is going to have any substance beyond being an eclectic collection of pictures that might have less coherence in them than the rest of an otherwise quite orderly life. I

D. N. Wheatley, *BipolART,*
DOI 10.1007/978-94-007-4872-9_11, © Springer Science+Business Media Dordrecht 2012

would describe myself as a person who prefers to have things organized both in my mind and surroundings. I have become perhaps less meticulous about this as I get older, partly as memory weakens. But I also do have what the clinical psychologist would call "unrelenting standards", a striving for having things in perfect order and trying to do all tasks to as high a standard as possible. There can be a quite frenetic desire to have everything clean and tidy, for example, in the kitchen or bathroom, which has often been a warning sign of an oncoming depression. Such frantic activity leads to poor motor co-ordination, with the result that I start dropping things. This is also a sign that makes me more irritable and I become increasingly aware of some forms of obsessional activity, involving trivial things like pointless counting, e.g. when putting cutlery away, measuring the number of steps it takes to get to the bottom of the garden, and noting how many strawberries I have just picked. I have sometimes stopped myself in mid-stream doing this, and then found after a similar interval has passed that I have a number in my head, as if I continued counting anyway. It turns out that the last number I had recorded seemingly unconsciously at the end of the task was about right. The proof of this has been on several occasions that I have carefully recounted all the items, and sure enough the final number tallied very closely indeed with the spontaneous counting (often only one or two out in a hundred, if not exactly the same).

Mental Stability in the General Public

The main confirmation of my mental health is from medical records stretching back to 1956 and what the doctors have thought of its severity, i.e. in relative terms on scales they might apply, e.g. the BSDS scale). On this basis, I have some disorder because of what BP does to disturb behaviour and body workings well away from the "norm". Norms themselves tell us very little if we do not know the degree of spread of values around them; in terms of the continuum from "normal" (euthymic) to mania or the other extreme, severe catatonic depression, we have no real idea how the general population is disposed along the spectrum. Leslie Weatherhead in *Psychology and Life* (1956) said *"Indeed, some of those (people) who are the most high-spirited and lighthearted seem, for that very reason, to be capable of going to the depths of depression."* Very many people on the continuum would never have subjected themselves to any form of assessment—they would seldom if ever admit to their condition let alone have its severity determined. This is well set out by Daniel Nettle in his book on *Strong Imagination–Madness, Creativity and Human Nature* (2001). In it he argues that he might be quite severely depressed, but he soldiers on because he has a high threshold for pain giving him the ability to put up with the discomfort, whereas his neighbour with far less severe symptoms but a low pain threshold is off work for 6 weeks. This shows that trying to place people on a spectrum is fraught with difficulties. This leads me to consider the plight of overly stressed business men and people in other taxing professions, many of whom may have mental problems that overtly are close to the manic and depressive states seen in a BP person, often writhing with *anxiety* and worry. The testosterone level on the busy stock exchange floor speaks volumes about the pressures we put ourselves under. Many people end up having a nervous breakdown, a colloquialism that is not itself a diagnosis in psychiatry. They are indeed "ill", whether they admit it or not.

> Love looks forwards, hate looks backward;
> anxiety has eyes all over its head.
>
> (Mignon McLaughlin)

None of us is mentally stable throughout a year, even less throughout life. Normality occurs sometimes in all of us, if that means a steady lifestyle with little stress (and perhaps not too much elation!). Some move from one extreme to another within a few minutes. We are all subject to swings of moods; but how many dare to admit how great these swings can be. Does my BP set me that much apart from most other people? On this basis, the answer is no; just that the swings are more noticeable to myself and others, and considerably more protracted, if not necessarily more extreme in intensity.

As the population becomes increasingly top heavy with regard to age, with ever more people living into their ninth and tenth (and even 11th) decades, mental illness will become one of the most prevalent disorders in mankind. One in six people will have been diagnosed as mentally ill, and that, as Roger Layard indicated (Layard, 2006), affects about one in three families in the country. The problem is exacerbated by the UK health system spending only 15% of its budget on mental illness, although it accounts for 50% of all the health problems. One in five people are likely to have dementia after the age of 65, i.e. unless something can be done about it, e.g finding ways stopping retireés from vegetating.

Depression affects the physiological functioning of the body; it makes you feel wretchedly ill (not so different from how some people feel mentally and physically when hit by a bad dose of virulent flu). One of the major difficulties that concerns the psychiatrists is not just the downturn in the general medical condition, but the question at almost every session of whether there has been any thought of "self-harm" (euphemistically implying—have you contemplated suicide"?). In my case, this has never seriously been considered; there has been no occasion over a 50 year period that I have contemplated any such act of self-harm. But I do know from my deep feelings that the time when this is most likely to happen is during the late stages of recovery when at times near manic surges and burst of energy occur, a time when irrational acts might occur. Knowing what is happening makes it much easier to get some control over one's state. This reminds me of the first dictum—"to know thyself!" and of a treasured quotation giving us an important lesson about life that was framed and hung in my bedroom as a child, given me at an very early age by one of my grandparents; it was *To Live* by Robert Louis Stevenson:

> We are all so busy and have so many far off projects to realise, we are in such haste to be doing, to be writing, to be gathering gear, that we forget that one thing of which these are but parts. Namely to live, to sit still and contemplate, to be everything and everywhere in sympathy, and yet content to remain where and what you are—is not this to know both wisdom and virtue, and dwell in happiness?

Art, Creativity and Its Place in Bipolar Disorder

What, in someone like myself with a life-long affliction with BP, is the effect not just on the mundane activities of daily living, but in my attempts to express myself in art? That is an extraordinarily difficult question to answer because you will have made your own subjective impression of my art. So how different is your subjective view from my subjective view? To sort out what is going on requires dialogue, and this would be valuable when reviewing this book with psychiatrists, clinical psychologists and related professionals, as well as people outside these health disciplines, especially friends and relatives (back to *Living with the black dog*).

In looking back on my life with BP, and particularly during the last 12–13 years, I am surprised at two things: first, having enough energy to accomplish many doodles and pictures when down; and second, in realising that creativity often springs from the gloom of depression as well as from euphoria. In the latter, enormous numbers of fascinating images are flooding into the mind that might easily be turned into pictures, but so many that they are lost as quickly as they come in, seldom if ever being captured and turned into art. They may, however, be stored in the memory and emerge during the depths of depression. Where do these ideas come from and does the BP sufferer have anything that might be considered an edge over the average person with regard to turning ideas into some form of reality—in making a greater than average contribution in some way or another (science, art, politics or whatever) to the sum total of human endeavour? There have been some indications that this is indeed the case, but being sceptical, I do not think the evidence is sufficiently convincing; or if it holds any water, it probably refers to a very small portion of the people who suffer from the disorder.

However, a recent study (see refs) at the Institute of Psychiatry in London has followed a number of previous investigations, and shown itself that there may indeed be some correlation. There is therefore only a little scientific evidence that creative people with strong imaginations excel in many walks of life from Generals to Poets have a higher incidence of BP than expected by chance. A similar notion is that an intense sex-drive heightens creative ability, but again I remain sceptical.

Taking things further, BP or manic depression has been linked with genius, not just creativity. The start of Brian Adam's book, *The Pits and the Pendulum* (2003), lists the names of many famous people who probably had BP disorder, and he begs the question—"so why me?" My own opinion is that if you visit places where people with BP meet regularly, you will find they come from all walks of life, but not necessarily that many are exceptionally talented or creative. If there are 6 million or more severe BP sufferers in the United States, there will probably be no clear bias towards more gifted individuals than would be expected by chance. However, some poets, such as Dryden, seem to think so, and he summed it up very succinctly, if we accept here that BP is indeed a form of "madness":

> Great wits are sure to madness near alli'd,
> And thin partitions do their bounds divide.
>
> (John Dryden: *Absolom and Achitophel*)

We met a similar expression in the opening quote of Aristotle in the Prologue. There is again a notion that creativity springs from where the imagination goes to extremes, and this is certainly true of manic-depression and other mental "aberrations". Some believe that the senses are duller during depression, but this is not true of the imagination, which can conjure up the most dreadful scenarios, as another poet John—in this case Milton—aptly wrote:

> Hence, loathed melancholy Of Cereberus, and blackest night born,
> In Stygian cave forlorn, 'Mongst horrid shapes, and shrieks, and sights unholy.
> (John Milton: *L'Allegro*)

A thought that has puzzled me for a long time concerns the nature of originality, of creativity. To put the question in perhaps its simplest form—can you dream up anything which your senses have not already encountered in some form or other? In brief, is there "anything new under the sun?" Are there inherently images that are given you by your hard-wiring, your inheritance, much like you can give expression to *instinctive behaviour* in other ways? However, these would amount to "preconceived" notions-again my scepticism does not make me believe in "memes", attributed to Dawkins (1989), but based on much earlier ideas of others, the name deriving from the Greek goddess of memory (Mnenosyne). Although you can think of a person with a normal human flesh-coloured face, it is not difficult to see in one's mind eye the same face with green or blue skin or grossly distorted in some other way. This comes down to variations on a theme, but can you have a truly original "theme"? Can you think "outside the box"? As Einstein remarked, to know something about the Universe, you have to step outside it (gedanken experiments). Can the imagination doing anything other than dressing up in almost infinitely different ways what one has already seen or heard from conception onwards? almost all Mythological creatures have been depicted as an amalgam of two known creatures—a griffon being an eagle head and a lion body. Perhaps some of the images found in scientific fiction come closer to "new" forms, but most nevertheless harp back to familiar forms. If we cannot be truly original, what I have been doing is regurgitating a whole plethora of mental images that have been built on existing themes concepts and images in my mind, but most of them dressed up in new guises.

> It is well established that much of our creative expression is birthed in the unconscious mind. To use creative expression and solutions in your everyday life, it is necessary to dip into the unconscious at will. Doodling is one way of doing this.
> (Henry Ward Beecher)

These may all have come from "impressions" gained throughout my life from birth (perhaps even before it). The brain is extraordinary in registering thousands of things that we think we have forgotten or simply committed to unconscious memory, as some new research on the brain seems to suggest—a question of whether we record everything that has ever impacted on our senses, at least when we wish to record things. A number of images in preceding chapters seem sometimes to have come from "out of nowhere", but they might just as easily simply recall impressions and images seen in my distant past (some have suggested previous lives, but my scepticism again means I am not going to be the kind of person to believe in reincarnation). Sam Kean in *The Disappearing Spoon* refers to eminent artists, e.g. van Gogh, Poe and William Crooks, concluding:

> Genius stems from parts of the psyche most of us cannot access, let alone harness for artistic purposes.

If the origin of ideas or images in art seems to be difficult to pin down, perhaps more can be learnt from looking at the situation from the scientific viewpoint on which I have more personal knowledge (and which will be discussed below). The doodle can start in a random way, but it becomes consolidated as more and more images appear in it of familiar objects, or at least suggest them. You (and others) begin to see things in the squiggles—just as you can look up at the clouds and see a face, a feather or a train.

The Influence of Others

The hard wiring and the memories indelibly written on the brain both mean that I lean on many others, as we all must do, who are living in the same times and world as myself, and others who have gone before me, regarding the way I respond to the world and, in this case, the way I have done so in producing my artwork. Perhaps the desired emotion or behaviour required to think outside the box is to question rather than accept what has gone before, and at times to be downright obstreperous (in the case of some artists, even to being obnoxious), to deliberately turn things upside-down and inside-out, to make ourselves and others see the worst in us, not just the sunnier side of life, which is often to get the message across as to how otherwise we might view the present state of affairs. They take stances and make comments on social, religious and political issues. If artists wear their hearts on their canvases rather than their sleeves, pictures clearly express powerful emotions, which might be seen as cathartic, a release valve of pent up feeling, the thing most needed in dispelling the angst and other feelings that trouble psychiatric patients. But does the majority of artwork derive from strong emotional expression? I can hardly believe that drawings of a bird or a plant as accurate reproductions of their form can be seen as an outpouring of emotion.

I have been interested throughout my life in art produced by many of the great masters, and there is no doubt that I have been seriously influenced by the outpourings of many of them, by whose standards I am a novice. In those that move you and me, it must be the emotional impact of their vision being passed on to the viewer. They have communicated powerfully at this level, and a silent dialogue has been opened.

A couple of instances in the pictures may help, par exemplum, to explain how I have leant on others in making my stance on similar subjects. One of my gravest—and yet to me, one of the most appealing—images is the one on page (presently), entitled *Falling into the Depths*. This moves from brighter red life-form motifs at the top to darker purple squares towards the bottom, in a gradual transition. There is no doubt that this piece echoes the sentiments of Mark Rothko, himself a sufferer who went from deep depression finally to suicide. But Rothko produced many of his "squares" over the years of his ever darkening mood. I used his basic theme and developed it within my own manner to produce this picture, but in the form of a composite without actually using squares—although they start to become so towards the bottom of the painting. Similarly, I leant heavily on Mondrian in the chapter on Geometry because I had a clear empathy with two of his elements, the first being the use of primary colours and the second his unwaving use of straight geometric lines (the rectilinear grid), which I thought might lend itself to some distortion in a space-time way. He seldom if ever used triangles or circles. I make no excuses for adopting and adapting the (style of the) artwork of others. It is hard not to copy others, especially where they have produced things that resonate well throughout mankind. I will take this argument a stage further, as mentioned above, in my role as a scientist. Indeed, being a researcher all my life, this is a career that demands creative thinking at all times.

Science—Its Relation to Art and Creativity

The scientist's main aim is to make some sense, an understanding, of Nature and the Universe through cause-effect. But everything is there, working as naturally as it ever has; we are not creating anything new in tangible terms. Biology was previously "Natural History", and took an almost purely descriptive approach. What the scientist does now is not just recapitulate what he sees (senses) and categorise (catalogue) it, but endeavours to make correlations. We begin to find out how things work and get a better the synthesis of the harmony of the Universe. Most people believe that science is highly sophisticated, making things very more complicated and difficult to understand. However, its main function is to make things simple, to explain things so that the layman can in turn begin to understand their significance. The whole edifice of scientific knowledge has been built up generation by generation not only on the "shoulders of giants", but on the backbone of hundreds of thousands of rank and file scientists and technologists who help in the important task of filling in the detail. The process of making direct and significant correlations demands "original thinking", even "lateral thinking", but not *out of the blue*, for in truth the whole structure is being constantly pieced together and the correlations that are important can suddenly become almost self-evident ("the penny drops"). An original thought that comes *completely* out of the blue is almost impossible to imagine. Perhaps art and science here are quite close to one another in thought-processing. In art, one is often striving to bring things together, to create an apposition that means something to others (that gets the message across), however facetious (e.g. *Ceci n'est pas un pipe*—by René Magritte).

The words of the Nobel Laureate, Albert Szënt-György, are very apt in this regard—"the gift is to see what everyone else sees, but think what no one else has thought," making new correlations that were never previously contemplated, for example that matter and energy are closely related, one being convertible into the other. New constructions can arise as a result, which might then lead to a complete unravelling of scientific problems (e.g. seeing the significance of the double helix of DNA in terms of genetics) or the development of new "schools" in art (those of the pointillists and cubists are obvious examples). How little difference in essence there is between the pixels of modern television monitors and the dots of Seurat's famous pictures!

Does it all matter? Creativity of the introspective artist—at some time, perhaps close to the end of life an artist may destroy much of his output. A lifetime of creation and devotion can go up in smoke in a few minutes. In science, individuality is not the issue in the long run; it is consensus that matters and therefore the edifice being built (usually by a series of ever advancing hypotheses) is passed on from generation to generation. However, let us read what Einstein had to say:

> After a certain level of technical skill is achieved, science and art tend to coalesce in aesthetics, plasticity and form. The greatest scientists are always artists as well.

Imagination

For people who do not have marked mood changes, life may be steady and imagination might not play an important part. It is not just the extreme difference in BP between the manic and the depressive moods, but the fact that during both moods the imagination is usually very active, from everything and anything been possible in the former, to the dark, bizarre, brooding and threatening pictures conjured up by the mind in deep depression, a point once again reiterated by Goldsmith.

> Don't let us make imaginary evils,
> when you know we have so many real ones to encounter
> (Oliver Goldsmith: *The Good-Natured Man*)

This remark echoes the sentiments of others about facing life, for example:

> We are more often frightened than hurt,
> and we suffer more from imagination than reality
> (The Dalai Lama: *The Art of Happiness*)

I would strongly support the notion that it is likely that BP sufferers will have a far more vivid imagination than the euthymic person. But in mania the imagination runs so fast that very few images can ever be caught and acted upon, at least during the "larger than life" episode. Most will be forgotten. In depression, the thoughts are often so morbid that it is difficult again to do anything about them; that is, unless there is a deliberate act of trying to capture some of these forms in words or pictures. This is why a doodle can be the germ of a major spontaneous drawing; it might go on to become something much grander, incorporating motifs that might have been lurking in the dark mind during depression.

It was only after all my doodling had been going for a long time, indeed quite recently, that I also became aware of the findings of Jackie Andrade (2010) that doodling has a definite place in memory recall. The question was posed whether doodling while listening to a telephone call helped or hindered recall of the content of a message. The results of a trial showed that the doodlers remembered 29% more information than the non-doodlers. But there is a remarkable finding that has received less recognition than the above, which is that the brain is more activity in boredom than when focused on a task. In greater free-wheeling in the former, the brain's computer strives to continue making lots of interconnections whereas the focused brain has less need to whirl around so freely. In earlier pages I have referred to the brain of the depressive also whirling around in useless rummaging, making one more exhausted than in the comparative clarity of the brain in mania. This is a quite unexpected, counterintuitive finding that may also shed a lot more light on the brain of the depressed patient.

As also mentioned earlier in the book, I never thought of myself as a doodler while listening to a lecture or a phone message, but this may have been due to the fact that I did have a very good (selectively eidetic) memory in my younger days. My notebooks, diaries, etc. seldom have doodles in them, so the one seen at the start of Chapter 2 that fell out of an old notebook was a surprise—I cannot recall now why I did this doodle (in fact I cannot even remember doing it, so some form of recall has little to do with this example!). Nevertheless, I can fully appreciate how information being sent to the brain can conjure up related or even tangential images that can lead to "spontaneous" drawing with a pen or pencil. But if there is not such a clear focus, the doodle might be a complete mish-mash, which could only be described as abstract. [Although I have titled many of mine as I indicated previously, many are so abstract and mixed up that there cannot be a descriptive title, i.e. one that can indicate the major features of the subject matter.] There are doodles in this book that are definitely the first of these types, the more recognisable in form, whereas the rest—perhaps the majority—are abstract. It is interesting that the early ones were more often depicting something (singular), although the finished article may not have been what was first in mind—it just ended up quickly that way as a variation on a basic item (a table, an urn, a flower). In contrast the more recently completed doodles have become increasingly larger, and are conglomerates of numerous motifs, shapes, shades and sizes that are much more random. There are few doodles that simply sprawl out in all directions; most are tidy and neat, now being kept within a firm outline in both cases. Interestingly, the later large doodles became increasingly contained within a rectangle, square or circle. I suggest this is a reflection of my "tidy mind"; tidiness is for me a bit of an obsession. When falling into depression, this becomes increasingly obvious. I start to be very particular about the cleanliness of a kitchen surface or a shower, in putting clothes away in the right draws and wardrobes, and other activities that have to be meticulously and often frenetically completed. The doodle, in releasing some of this inner tension should have a useful preventive role in BP, but I did not use it until very recently as an aid to defusing the possibility of sliding into depression. In recent times, starting to doodle has become increasingly important and can be helpful in quietening the mind, especially before retiring to bed. If it is true for me, perhaps it might work for others, and I sincerely hope this is the case. I have no idea why it took me so long to learn this lesson.

One of the benefits of doodling as opposed to setting out to draw or paint a precise picture (for example, all the thousands called "still life") is that there is no need to consider anything a mistake. If you are not satisfied with some part, you can simply scribble all over it or change it into some different form. This is why the outcome of a doodle is almost always unpredictable. It is highly adaptable as a spontaneous artform. A doodle unfolds as each segment/squiggle is done; but as it develops it usually suggests what to do next. The bits may be disparate, but in some cases a theme starts to emerge, such as "Leviathan" on page (39). In others, it is sometimes seas, ships, hills, and animals; but you have seen them already and can find things or themes in them that I do not!

Is the elaborate doodle a serious art-form—has the finished product any place in the wider world of art? That is something for you to decide. Where is the dividing line between an elaborate doodle and a large abstract painting, as might have been done by established artists of note, perhaps someone like Wassily Kandinsky.

Anger and Bipolar Disorder

There can be anger in BP; in some it becomes uncontainable and can be distressing for those closest to the sufferer. There is anger in the frustration of falling into depression, and there is anger during the later stages of recovery when energy returns and things are attempted before the mind and body are functioning in sufficient harmony. Is this anger reflected in the doodles or pictures? I do not think that the artwork I have shown has much anger pent up in them; if they were calming my mind, then anger was being dissipated, not being pent up and released explosively—as might otherwise have happened, like the wild burst of a activity caught on canvas in the pictures of Jackson Pollock. I cannot remember being angry when producing any of my pictures, although there was huge frustration in doing the large abstract called "Two spheres" in the chapter on Abstraction (75), probably because it was done in short bursts of painting during and after a severe depression, and took ages to come together, unlike so many other pictures. In contrast some have been completed with astonishing speed.

The originality in my pictures may not be that great, but the doodles are examples of the mind free-wheeling, or so I would like to think. That all depends on what constraints are operating behind the level of the conscious when one is "free-wheeling". The elements of some of the more elaborate doodles in the early chapters might all be reproductions of images ingrained in my mind since infancy, but they have also been juxtaposed in some way—whether it is ordered or quite random is difficult to know. It is these, and their extensions regarding in particular the pictures found in the chapters on Abstract and Geometry, and therefore we need to consider what is happening in terms of the mind, art and therapy.

Doodling—A Natural Approach to Art Therapy

Some psychologists suggest that doodling has its place in our lives—that it is not just an idle or indeed a useless activity. It is worth going into more detail about these findings because, if the ideas do hold water, the role of doodling as an art-form in therapy might be more fully explored—it might even prove important. If doodles are a kind of free-wheeling activity, this is perhaps the way in which the trapped mind of the depressed BP sufferer (as for other mental disorders) can be released from the worst of the symptoms (see Table 11.1 that follows). Art therapy might benefit greatly from these preliminary investigations, brought more clearly into the public domain by studies like those of Jackie Anrade mentioned above, but from inklings that had previously been put forward by several other psychologists. A doodle portrays an image that acts as a symbol to make the recall of a telephone conversation, a lecture or some other form of communication easier. Many people with phenomenal memories do not just remember what they have seen or heard; each element to be stored in the memory seems to be attached to some kind of visual image and these images form a sequence that helps the next element to be recalled, and so on. This was precisely the case with the famous patient "S" of Alexander Luria (1987), who purportedly remembered everything he had ever read verbatim. In brief, doodling can be a useful functions in daily life and its use by people with mental disorders might find that doodling is not only a release in allowing expression to occur, but gets the mind into better order (reduces confusion).

From my own experience, I feel sure that doodling is helpful, therapeutic and not a waste of time. It can take its place in art therapy, and can almost certainly be honed to much greater advantage than suggested here. This feeling seems to be confirmed by two observations; first, in more recent times I have produced far more (and more elaborate) doodles during depression than previously. And second, I have begun to find that if I start doodling before I perceive that I am sinking into depression, it seems to ameliorate some of the symptoms of its onset—it may act in a preventive way, which is perhaps bring out its true value.

Features of Depression

> Manic depression distorts moods and thoughts, incites dreadful behaviours, destroys the basis of rational thought, and too often erodes the desire and the will to live.
> I have become fundamentally and deeply sceptical that anyone who does not have this illness can truly understand it.
>
> (Kay Redfield Jamison: *An Unquiet Mind*)

The (mental) sickness of all mankind in these days when everyone for some reason seems to have to rush around (lunch US style—"grab n' go"). The borderline between stress leading to nervous exhaustion and a general depressive state, but not necessarily of clinical severity, cannot easily be decided by psychiatrists and clinical psychologists. Attention has been drawn that suggests that many TV, movie and celebrity characters epitomise states of mental disorder. Suicide rates are high in celebrities who dash around the world under constant physical and mental stress. It is no wonder they try to "opt out" by resorting to drugs.

The one thing about BP, especially its depressive state, is that I would not wish it on my worst enemy. But as Kay Redfield Jamison (1955) remarked, she was for a long time reluctant to be "normal" because of the excitement and vividness of life in the manic state. It is as if one pays the price of this joyousness by having to put up with the opposite.

The worst features (the words *symptoms* and *characteristics* would do equally well) of depression can probably be summed up in the categories that are listed in the following table.

Table 11.1

Type of function affected	Condition
Physiological	Excessive tiredness
	Listlessness/low ebb of physical energy
	Tight throat
	Headaches (often frontal oppression)
	Nausea
	Bad breath
	Dry and dull hair, poor skin condition
	Poor coordination
	"Hot" nerves, e.g. across shoulders
	Loss of libido
	Loss of appetite
	Feeling as of irritable bowel syndrome
Psychological	Deep anxiety
	Desperation and panic
	Lack of concentration
	Poor memory recall
	Irritability
	Deep suspicion of other peoples' behaviour
	Obsessional thoughts
	Loss of self-esteem
	Loss of confidence
	Poor and restless sleep*
	Photophobia
	Lack of "reality" of familiar objects
	Acute awareness of self
	Loss of expression of emotions
	Inability to make decisions
Social	Need for isolation, introversion
	Avoidance of anything unfamiliar
	Avoidance of anything threatening (e.g. crowds)
	Inability to cope with adverse events (e.g. bereavement)
	Inability to interact socially and reciprocate feeling of others
	Desire to stay in bed, avoid daily routine
	Slow and poor communication

*A note of sleep. Sleep is so important in both the depressive and manic phases of BP—or at least good rest. But the torment of the former or the exuberance of the latter gives little opportunity of getting proper sleep.

These are the ones I have noted myself and are probably experienced by the majority of BP sufferers. It is not an exhaustive list, but it is long enough for anyone to appreciate the way in which in the down phase of BP (and monopolar) depression totally envelopes the body as well as the mind; it is a completely pervasive disorder.

To be uncomfortable in the body is one thing, but to be uncomfortable in mind as well moves human experience into a different dimension that makes it truly difficult to bear. During depression, the mind becomes very aware of the body—you might listen anxiously, wondering whether your heart is beating properly, and the nausea and churning of the stomach can be worse to abide than the oppressive frontal headaches.

> The worst of depression lies in a present moment that cannot escape from the past it idealises or deplores.
>
> (Andrew Solomon: *The Noonday Demon*)

> O magic sleep! O comfortable bird!
> That broodest o'er the troubled sea of the mind
> Till it is hushed and smoothed!
>
> (John Keats)

In Touch with Infinity, Unity, God

There is a notion that the mind can be lost when it is not "in touch" with infinity—the idea that there is some relationship with eternity and that life is not a totally transient experience, but this is an idea in which I personally have little belief. It is an odd concept that suggests that the human being might see himself or herself as having a place within a continuum of the existence of the Universe. Being in touch with "reality", whatever that is to each of us, is an important aspect of life that gets badly disturbed in BP disorder and many other mental health conditions. Reality, much as our understanding of things in science, comes through consensus. If we move too far from the consensus as individuals, we lose touch with that which is common to all human society; we can become entirely isolated, alienated, stigmatized and possibly outlawed, although we tend to take these steps ourselves. There is no question that between the manic and depressive states, the "normal" being has a strong sense of a more stable "reality", the tangible nature of the environment, in which we live. In the severely depressed state, this is very noticeably changed; almost nothing accords with the "normal" recollection of things that was the situation beforehand; everything can indeed become alien and strange. The unfamiliarity of things plus the fact that one cannot handle anything physically or emotionally with even the least degree of aptitude quickly makes the ethos unbearable, and quite abhorrent—out of touch with reality, even the reality you had previously created—the condition prevalent in so many mental disorders. From being a part of your world, you suddenly have lost that feeling of unity and involvement, and then the isolation that follows is dreaded, and then dreadful as it arrives. The irony is that in many respects you desperately want this isolation ("leave me alone, please shut out the world!"), but you also know that you need the warmth of humanity to survive. These two states fight with one another, bringing the torment of severe depression to a head; depression is a time of huge conflict in the brain, the negative fighting the weak positive thoughts most of the time (the innate will to live). The brain is very active, more so in its confusion than during euthymic periods.

The change from one state to the other can be startling fast, extremely frightening, and quite devastating. It has happened within a few minutes, as in one episode (at the start of October 2009) when I leant against the kitchen table and looked at my partner early one evening and said "I'm going". Five or 10 minutes later I was in a very bad state, which unfortunately continued for well over 3 months. There had not been any clear warning signs on that occasion before beginning to feel low. I might have been quite manic for several months, but that mania did not seem out of control. [I take mood stabilising drugs daily—lithium does not work for me—but I have no real notion that they make any significance difference.] The most capable of people can often suffer the most debilitating depressions in which they accuse themselves of being utterly incapable of anything. To such a person, the change is usually devastating. These highly contrasting viewpoints (called "moods") will be occurring throughout depressive episodes, not only on these matters I have just discussed, but on a whole range of other issues, from the smallest details being blown out of all proportion to the very struggle with the big questions about such things as one's mortality and very existence. Obsessional thoughts take over, from the trivial to the profound. In depression, the id has tried to withdraw completely and very little can now be externalised, although there are other BP sufferers unlike myself who vent their negativity in a destructive show of considerable force.

> Everything previously moving with the grain is now against it—you are irritable, angry, frightened, uncontrollable, and enmeshed totally in the blackest caves of the mind. You never knew those caves were there. It will never end, for madness carves its own reality
>
> (Kay Redfield Jamison: *An Unquiet Mind*)

To do so requires enough emotional and physical energy to externalise oneself seemingly against all odds, and I have always found this impossible. My experience is that only during the later stages of recovery might this happen, when irritability becomes increasingly manifest. In terms of physical activity, this would be akin to undertaking a prize-fight with yourself, knowing how senseless and futile this would be. Is this the basis of self-harming?

In hypomania, one is tumbling over oneself in taking reality beyond it sensible bounds, believing that in this world things are bigger and better than anyone else can imagine until one gets totally out of touch with what others consider normality by consensus.

In dealing with depression, it is certainly a good thing to take plenty of exercise (e.g. long walks) to raise the levels of the endorphins, but the first step is the hardest to take. Returning to obsessional thoughts, this is indeed true of both depression and mania, except that in the former one has just a few very deep and black ones, while in mania you can be overwhelmed by obsessional thoughts of projects that just have to be followed through, each piling on one another, as if there were time to give them all maximum attention and yet expect to manage every one of them to fruition.

Meditation on the theme of the unity of everything needs to be recommended to most BP sufferers, but this is not an easy business. It calls for a high degree of self-discipline. Outside the low periods, the desire may be strong enough to start disciplining oneself, but as soon as the low comes, it is quite a different matter. Taking this one step further, the notion of the unity of all things and the harmony of the universe may be ascribed not to its intrinsic nature, but to the hand of God. The universe is here because it is the creation of a deity. This is a troublesome subject which I, as an agnostic/atheist, do not wish to dwell on in any way, other than to say that BP sufferers seem to have much the same experiences whether they are believers or not. But I am also of the persuasion that if there is a train of thought that can help relieve the depressed "soul" or quieten the actions of manic episodes, then belief in God, or what you will, may be a very useful crutch. When despair is writ large across the brow, the "soul" (for which read id) is truly grasping at straws, for any small thing that will lessen the pain and lift the deadness brought about by what Andrew Solomon calls the "noonday demon". Let The Dalai Lama (1998) give us again some of his wisdom in dealing with one of the most human of emotions that sadly gets squashed out of existence in much of the hurly-burly of modern day life:

> Compassion is not religious business, it is human business, it is not a luxury, it is essential for our own peace and mental stability, it is essential for human survival.

Psychology tells us about the process of *thought transference*, which seems to me to be relevant in this context. If you can put your soul, your faith, truly in the hands of God, then the believer has something which might be helpful in getting the depressed out of what Bunyan referred to as the "slough of despond". But we all seem to be doing this, whether we are BP or normal. If you do not try to put yourself in the mind of Mozart, El Greco or Frank Sinatra, you will not get from others the inspiration and motivation that is needed to do anything. To play Mozart well you have to think Mozart (as if you were he). We rely heavily on the ideas of others in order to have ideas of our own, and something that is lacking during depression is the inability to be "inspired" to do anything, to shun role-models. Oddly, and tangentially, this leads me to another helpful ploy. The word "inspired" is exactly the same as used medically for the taking in of breath. Coming round full circle, we are reliably informed by people in many walks of life, from doctors to gurus, that living is all about breathing. Few of us discipline ourselves in how to breathe properly. A great deal of bodily relaxation can come from proper exercise of the lungs. This also goes along with regular exercise of the whole of the body, indulging in steady activities such as swimming or walking. Relief from depression comes via many different channels, each of which will affect the healthiness of our body and mind. If depression was purely a chemical disturbance in the brain, then an effective remedy would have been found long ago. If there is a major genetic component to it through inheritance, then it might be sensible to search for the genes responsible, if they could be pinned down to a manageable few—Kay Redfield Jamison mentions that this is the quest of Jim Watson (of double helix fame), much as Francis Crick was particularly intrigued in his later life to know the genetic basis and molecular biology of memory. But it is not; depression affects the whole of one's being (see the Table 11.1). Correction of some brain chemistry is needed, with some people responding for example to lithium, but there are most definitely natural substances in the brain that can make one euphoric rather than depressed. Natural "endorphins" or unnatural drugs of this kind can help to make the immediate situation more acceptable than being purely in a vegetative state. This last expression conjures up to me quite a lot of the nature of the depressive phase of BP disorder. It takes a multifaceted approach to get to grips with the treatment of BP disorder; but it can have so many "faces" that it is unlikely that a general "therapeutic" approach will be found that can help the greater majority of sufferers.

A mind enlightened is like heaven; a mind in darkness is hell
(Chinese proverb)

And the Future?

Will mental stress increase to the point of needing medical intervention in an ever increasing proportion of the aging population? Undoubtedly this will be the case unless steps are taken to reduce the "work" ethic—the stress-based sickness that is driven by competition, consumerism, greed and selfishness. We may be living longer, but at a price, with the proportion of people over 65 developing Alzheimer's or dementia increasing considerably not only as a percentage but in absolute numbers, creating a massive problem needing to be addressed now rather than wait any longer. It is no fun to be living 20 years longer on average if these years are going to be marred by more and more mental illness. Will we be able to prevent the manic-depressive from going to extremes? How will this impact on the creativity of mankind—would it make the slightest difference? One can only conclude that for those who from time to time are locked away in the deep depression of BP, it is a truly unpleasant condition. It needs to be alleviated and preferably by some intervention that does not make the sufferer a zombie for months at a time. The use of art therapy could be widened, and within it I would hope my contribution in recommending doodling can offer an inroad that people will recognise as having some potential, as indicated in Chapter 3 and elsewhere. Within that chapter, I refer to several studies and books that deal with, even extol, the virtues of "spontaneous drawing"/doodling in psychotherapy. I now endorse the views of these scientists and doctors who believe that this is playing—or should be playing—a major role in helping prevent depression as much as getting out of it.

I can look back now at a large "gallery" of artwork that I have created over the last 12–13 years and feel satisfied in several ways. First, I am quite overwhelmed by the products of my efforts that were made when I would for most of the time be classed as clinically unwell. Second, that I have more recently developed a particular style of doodle that seems in many ways unique, a genre in a manner of speaking. And third, that without any further formal training in art, I now seem to accomplish some things with considerably more expertise. While this might be seen as rather self-patronizing—which it admittedly is!—one of the things that the depressive cannot do is indulge in self-adulation, but almost invariably the opposite, self-deprecation. However, when you have successfully used your skill and practices to avoid falling into the extremes of BP, you do deserve to pat yourself on the back and say well done. There is light at the end of the tunnel. If this book has interested you in the art done by someone with BP, then it is worth remembering what one wag once said:

> Art never expresses anything but itself
>
> (Oscar Wilde: *The Decay of Living*)

References

Adams B (2003) The Pits and the Pendulum: A Life With Bipolar Disorder. Jessica Kingsley Publishers, London

Agutter PS, Wheatley DN (2008) About life. Springer, Dordrecht

Andrade J (2010) What does Doodling Do? Appl Cognitive Psych 24:100-106

BPDS at www.psychiatrictimes.com/clinical-scales/bsds

Carr C (2007) Living with the Black Dog: How to Cop When Your Partner is Depressed. White Ladder Press, (now Crimson Publishers), Richmond

Dawkins R (1989) The Selfish Gene. Oxford University Press, Oxford (Refers to "memes", Inherited Memory Traces, a Hypothesis with Little Evidence to Support it; The Word Based on Mnemosyne, Greek Goddess of Memory.)

Dean S (2010) The Disappearing Spoon. Hachette Books Group US, New York

Exner JE, Rorschach H (2002) The Rorschach: Basic Foundations and Principles, vol 1. Wiley and Sons, USA

Harding DE (1986) On Having No Head: Zen and the Rediscovery of the Obvious. Arkana, London

HH Dalai Lama, Butler HC (1998) The Art of Happiness. Riverhead, New York

Henson J (2010) Doodling with Jim Henson: More than 50 Fun and Fanciful Exercises to Inspire the Doodler in you. Walter Fortes, USA

Institute of Psychiatry at www.independent.co.uk/news/science/you-dont-have-to-be-a-genius-ndash-but-it-helps-1887646.html (a news item on research to be published from the Institute of Psychiatry in London along with Swedish colleagues from Stockholm)

Jamison KR (1955) An Unquiet Mind. AA Kopf Ltd., New York

Kyaga S, Lichenstein P, Boman M, Hultman C, Landström N, Landén M (2011) Creativity and Mental Disorder: Family Study of 300,000 People with Severe Mental Disorder. Brit J Psychiat 199:373-379

Layard R (2006) The Depression Report—a New Deal for Depression and Anxiety Disorders http://rep/lse.ac.uk/textonly/research/mentalhealth/DEPRESSION_REPORT_LAYARD-pdf

Luria A (1987) The Mind of a Mnemonist: A Little Book About a Vast Memory. Harvard University Press, Cambridge

Mansfield E (2008) The Little Book of the Mind. Lovely Little Books, Plymouth

Nettle D (2001) Strong Imagination—Madness, Creativity and Human Nature. Oxford University Press, Oxford

Solomon A (2001) The Noonday Demon. Catto and Windus, London

Weatherhead L (1957) Psychology and Everyday Life. Hodder and Stoughton, London

Wheatley DN (1982) The Centriole: A Central Enigma of Cell Biology. Elsevier North Holland, Amsterdam

D. N. Wheatley, *BipolART,*
DOI 10.1007/978-94-007-4872-9,

Index

D. N. Wheatley, *BipolART*,
DOI 10.1007/978-94-007-4872-9, © Springer Science+Business Media Dordrecht 2012

MIX
Papier aus verantwortungsvollen Quellen
Paper from responsible sources
FSC® C105338

If you have any concerns about our products,
you can contact us on
ProductSafety@springernature.com

In case Publisher is established outside the EU,
the EU authorized representative is:
Springer Nature Customer Service Center GmbH
Europaplatz 3, 69115 Heidelberg, Germany

Printed by Libri Plureos GmbH
in Hamburg, Germany